Nurse to Nurse
WOUND CARE

Nurse to Nurse
WOUND CARE

Donna Scemons, RN, FNP-BC, MSN, MA, CNS, CWOCN
President, Healthcare Systems, Inc.
Family Nurse Practitioner, Wound, Ostomy, and Continence Care

Denise Elston, RN, BSN, CWOCN
Consultant, Private Practice
Wound, Ostomy and Continence Care for Acute Care, Outpatient,
  Home Health, Hospice and Long Term Care

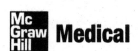 **Medical**

New York Chicago San Francisco Lisbon London Madrid Mexico City
New Delhi San Juan Seoul Singapore Sydney Toronto

The **McGraw·Hill** Companies

Nurse to Nurse: Wound Care

2 3 4 5 6 7 8 9 0   DOC/DOC   12 11 10 9

Set ISBN 978-0-07-149397-0; MHID 0-07-149397-2
Book ISBN 978-0-07-159079-2; MHID 0-07-159079-X
PDA card ISBN 978-0-07-159080-8; MHID 0-07-159080-3

This book was set in Berkeley Book by International Typesetting and Composition.
The editor was Quincy McDonald.
The production supervisor was Catherine H. Saggese.
Project management was provided by Preeti Longia Sinha of International
Typesetting and Composition.
The designer was Eve Siegel.
The cover designer was David Dell'Accio.
RR Donnelley was printer and binder.

This book is printed on acid-free paper.

Library of Congress Cataloging-in-Publication Data

Scemons, Donna.
  Nurse to nurse. Wound care / Donna Scemons, Denise Elston.
    p. ; cm.
  Includes bibliographical references and index.
  ISBN 978-0-07-149397-0 (pbk. : alk. paper)
  1. Wounds and injuries—Nursing. I. Elston, Denise. II. Title.
 III. Title: Wound care.
  [DNLM: 1. Wounds and Injuries—nursing. WY 154 S289n 2009]
  RD93.95.S34 2009
  617.1—dc22

                     2008015169

*This book is dedicated to all the patients, caregivers,
family members, CWOCNs, educators, nurses,
physical therapists, physicians, and other healthcare professionals
who have taught and encouraged us throughout our professional
careers. Without these shoulders to stand on this book would
not have been possible. In this, it is our sincerest hope that other
healthcare professionals will find this text useful
in their clinical endeavors.*

Contents

Acknowledgments

This book would not have been possible without the support and understanding of Robin, Gaetano, Samuel, Jason, and my partner in this endeavor, Denise Elston.

DS

Thank you Bill, Goldine, Leslie, and Donna Scemons for your support. And in memory of my father, Martin P. Elston, MD, thank you for providing inspiration to me.

DE

Thanks also to all the fine individuals at McGraw-Hill who worked diligently with fledgling authors, were always encouraging, and confident that this could and would be completed.

DS and DE

List of Acronyms

AAI	Ankle/arm index
ABI	Ankle brachial index
ACE	American Association of Clinical Endocrinologists
ADA	American Diabetic Association
ADLs	Activities of daily living
AHRQ	Association for Healthcare Research and Quality
ASO	Arteriosclerosis obliterans
BP	Blood pressure
CHF	Congestive heart failure
CLT	Complex lymphedema therapy
CPDT	Complex physical decongestive therapy
CPT	Complex physical therapy
CVI	Chronic venous insufficiency
DVT	Deep venous thrombosis
EGF	Epidermal growth factor
ESR	Erythrocyte sedimentation rate
FGF	Fibroblast growth factor
HBO	Hyberbaric oxygen
ILD	Indentation load deflection
IL-1	Interleukin-1
LDL	Low-density lipoprotein
MLD	Manual lymph drainage
MODS	Multiple organ dysfunction syndrome
NPUAP	National Pressure Ulcer Advisory Panel
NS	Normal saline
OT	Occupational therapist
PAN	Polyarteritis nodosa
PAOD	Peripheral arterial occlusive disease
PDGF	Platelet-derived growth factor
PN	Polyarteritis nodosa
POC	Plan of care
PT	Physical therapist
PTSD	Post-traumatic stress disorder
PV	Pemphigus vulgari
PVD	peripheral vascular disease

RBC	Red blood cell
RN	Registered nurse
ROM	Range of motion
SLE	Systemic lupus erythematosus
TBSA	Total body surface area
TGF-β	Transforming growth factor-beta
VLDL	Very-low-density lipoprotein
WBC	White blood cell
WOCN	Wound ostomy continence nurse

Nurse to Nurse
WOUND CARE

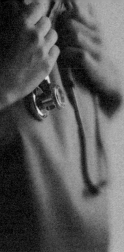

Chapter 1

ETHICAL CONSIDERATIONS IN WOUND EVALUATION AND MANAGEMENT

 KEY POINTS

- The ethical concepts discussed are presented from a western perspective.
- Application of ethical principles is necessary for any and all wound management.
  - The role of ethics in wound management
- Ethics and ethical behavior including:
  - Paternalism
  - Autonomy
  - Beneficence
  - Nonmaleficence
  - Fidelity
  - Role fidelity
  - Veracity
  - Conflict of interest
  - Confidentiality
  - Justice
- Potential internet resources

THE ROLE OF ETHICS IN WOUND CARE

Performing an evaluation, assessment, or management of any type of wound is an ethical endeavor and may present ethical challenges at times. In this chapter, the ethical principles and concepts within Western health care—most commonly known as biomedical ethics (the ethics of health-care)—will be discussed. The specific concepts of paternalism, autonomy, beneficence, nonmaleficence, fidelity, role fidelity, veracity, therapeutic privilege, conflict of interest, confidentiality, and justice will be addressed. It is important to note that the concepts herein are viewed from a Western perspective, and the wise health-care provider acknowledges this and provides care in a culturally aware manner.

The area of wound management provides an opportunity for the patient, the family, and caregivers to acknowledge aspects of their lives that otherwise may never have been addressed with any health-care provider. Some of the areas that may be discussed are beliefs about health, illness, and healing; the cause of the wound; and what the patient and family think will heal the wound, or even if they believe the wound will heal. In addressing these topics, the health-care provider may experience a single culture or belief system or a mixture of one or more cultures and belief systems.

The privilege of professional access to the patient, the family, and caregivers brings with it certain moral obligations or moral duties. It is important for the nurse to consider the concept of morals which in essence means the general "principles of right and wrong in relation to human actions and character."[1]

The Nurse's Ethical Duty

The nurse might wonder why consideration of morals is of any importance when what he or she is doing is providing clinical services for some type of wound. The practice of wound care is fraught with areas in which the morals or society's determination of right and good conduct of the health-care professional may be seriously tested. Understanding the concepts of morals, moral duty, and moral obligation are critical in providing wound care.

The privilege of professional access to patients brings specific obligations and duties, including the following:

- The patient's interests are placed above the personal interest of the nurse. If this duty is overlooked or forgotten, the contract (standard of practice) among the health-care provider, the health-care organization, and the patient is broken.

  — Example: The health-care provider conducts a seminar and needs wound photographs to supplement the written and verbal components of the presentation. The provider takes photographs of the patient's wounds solely for the purpose of using them in the seminar. The only reason for taking these photographs is for the convenience of the health-care provider, and therefore the activity is actually for the nurse's personal interest and not for the patient's best interest. To avoid any consideration that the photographs are for personal interest, the patient would need to grant the nurse informed consent to use the photographs. The nurse would need to assure the patient that any refusals on the patient's part would have no effect on the nurse-patient relationship or the patient's treatment.

- The patient's privacy is protected from another individual's or society's desire to know details of the patient's treatment.

  — Who has the legal right to know about the patient's wound?

  — What is the health-care provider's responsibility in this? This differs somewhat from state to state and country to country. It is the health-care provider's responsibility to have a complete understanding of the legal rights of all involved.

— Who does not have the legal right to know about the patient's condition? What is the health-care provider's responsibility in this? Once again, it is ultimately the responsibility of the nurse to know the legal rights of the patient, family, and health-care provider. However, in many areas of the world, the general public does not have any legal right to knowledge concerning the patient's care, progress, or prognosis. The health-care provider must identify if the health-care organization has a policy or procedure concerning this challenge. If such a policy or procedure is available, it is generally considered appropriate for the health-care provider to acknowledge and follow these mandates.

Remember

Assess each organization's policy and procedure concerning confidentiality before providing information about a specific patient to anyone other than another health-care provider who will be providing evaluation or treatment to the patient.

· Does the health-care provider have a duty to treat the patient who has a wound(s)?
— There is no one correct answer to this question, but guidelines do exist. In general, most health-care professions have created a "code of ethics" for referral when a member has an ethical question. As an example, the American Nurses Association (ANA) has published guidelines to assist nurses in determining if a moral *duty* for treatment exists, or if it is merely a moral *option*.
— The criteria for making this type of decision include:
  1. The patient is at significant risk of harm, loss, or damage if the practitioner does not assist in treatment.

2. The practitioner's intervention or care is directly relevant to preventing harm.

3. The practitioner's care will probably prevent harm, loss, or damage to the patient.

4. The benefit the patient will gain outweighs any harm the practitioner might incur and does not present more than a minimal risk to the health-care provider.[2]

According to the ANA, if the answer to all four criteria is *yes*, it would be considered a moral duty for the nurse to treat the patient under the principle of beneficence. However, if all four criteria could not be answered in the affirmative, the decision to treat would become a moral option and not a moral duty. It is important to remember that this information concerns the ethical decision making only and is not to be construed as presenting a legal argument for or against treatment. Failure to treat may have potential legal consequences.

Remember

Review the code of ethics specific to the health-care provider's clinical discipline whenever concerns or questions arise that may be of an ethical nature.

ETHICS AND ETHICAL BEHAVIOR

Ethics and ethical behavior are based on moral attitudes and moral conduct, not on legal precedents. The moral purpose of wound care is to preserve and/or improve healing, and to preserve and/or improve the patient's or caregiver's independence.

The ethical decisions that occur in wound care are often referred to as ethical dilemmas. One example is

- Under various reimbursement sources the decision has been made that only a specified amount of money may be applied to patients with wounds, or

- Specific amounts of treatment are authorized for patients with wounds (e.g., a limited number of encounters or visits), or

Another example would be:

- Only specified types or brands of wound products are available for patients with wounds, or
- Specific levels of health-care providers are authorized to provide care based solely on monetary reasons.

The dilemma faced by the health-care provider is deciding what is better for the individual patient, and does the duty exist to provide care or products that may not be reimbursable. There is no single, correct answer to this ethical dilemma.

Each situation must be evaluated and weighed on its own merits. When faced with such decisions, the health-care provider may choose to request the assistance of an ethics committee, an ethicist, or another health-care provider with more experience in dealing with these types of ethical dilemmas. Some reflection on the concept of paternalism would also be helpful for the health-care provider faced with what he or she considers an ethical dilemma.

Paternalism

Paternalism as a term has been dated from the 1880s by the *Oxford English Dictionary* as meaning "the principle and practice of paternal administration; government as by a father; the claim or attempt to supply the needs or to regulate the life of a nation or community in the same way a father does those of his children." Due to the reference to a father, it would seem that paternalism creates a situation in which one person acts like a father to or for another, and in doing so makes decisions about health-care rather than allowing the individual to make his or her own decisions. This was in fact the method used for several centuries by many health-care providers. The health-care provider knew what was best for the patient and therefore selected the specific action without consideration for the patient's decision-making ability. Additionally, there is generally some type of coercion or force involved on the part of the health-care provider in the presence of paternalism. More insidious methods that may be seen as paternalistic involve deception, dishonesty, nondisclosure of information, partial disclosure of information, or manipulation of information with the intent of unduly influencing the patient or caregiver's decision.

It is true that as a health-care provider it is an expectation that the provider has superior knowledge, education, and insight about the patient's wound and overall health. Therefore, the health-care provider has a special fiduciary relationship with the patient and is in an authoritative position in which he or she is expected to know more about the wound, wound treatments, and so forth than the patient. However, from a Western perspective, the health-care provider must not interfere with or refuse to conform to the patient's choices regarding his or her welfare.

According to Beauchamp and Childress, paternalism is "the intentional overriding of one person's known preferences or actions by another person, where the person who overrides justifies the action by the goal of benefiting or avoiding harm to the person whose preferences or actions are overridden."[2] In wound care, it is of significant importance for the health-care provider to explain thoroughly everything to the patient and caregiver, allow them time to ask questions, and allow them the opportunity to make appropriate decisions relative to treatment type, location, time frames, and expected outcomes. These actions allow the patient to make autonomous decisions concerning wound management.

Autonomy

In health-care, the term autonomy may be used with the concept of self-determination. It literally means that the patient or designee has the freedom to choose and implement that choice. It presupposes that the patient or designee has the intellectual competence and power to make treatment decisions. For the health-care provider, it means that all available information has been provided to the patient, caregiver, and or designee without deception, dishonesty, nondisclosure of information, partial disclosure of information, or manipulation of information. It also means that the health-care provider respects the autonomy of others (patient, caregiver, or designee).

Practicing wound management in a multicultural society requires the health-care provider to continually update his or her knowledge and understanding about the concept of autonomy in cultures different from the provider's. For example, in many tribal societies decisions about treatment can only be made after thorough discussion with the patient's community. Such discussion may take several hours to several days depending on the location of the patient, the location of the treatment center, and the patient's community. Additionally, it is the patient who determines what is meant by community. It is entirely possible that to a specific patient community means the entire group or tribe and may or may not have spiritual connotations.

It is under this ethical concept that the health-care provider's obligation to make disclosure is found. Using legal terms, this translates to the principle of informed consent; however, in more ethical terms, informed consent indicates that the patient or designee has substantial understanding of the proposed wound management and has not been forced or coerced into authorizing the nurse or health-care professional to provide specific care or treatment. Therefore, the health-care provider should ask these questions when determining that the patient or designee has agreed to the proposed wound management program.

- Does the patient or designee have the competence to understand the provided health-care information and to make a decision based on this information?
- Has the patient or designee voluntarily offered his or her consent for this wound management program without fear of or actual force or coercion?
- Was the disclosure of information provided which could be considered material to a decision of agreeing to or refusing this management plan?
- Was all the information the health-care provider believes is significant, presented?

- Was there a specific management plan explained including expected time frames and outcomes?
- Was there a decision for or against the specific management plan?
- Did the patient or designee actually authorize the specific wound management plan?

Remember

Assess the organization's policy and procedures concerning ethics referrals whenever there are concerns or questions about a patient's autonomy or competence.

Beneficence

Beneficence refers to the ethics principle indicating a moral obligation to "act for the benefit of others."[2] For the health-care provider involved in wound management, beneficence is a duty to promote the health and welfare of the patient by honoring the patient's autonomy. For the wound management patient, it also means:

- Wound treatments should have a positive effect on the healing process, NOT simply create no regression in the healing process.
- All wound management activities are done to promote the patient's best interests.
- The health-care provider works to actively remove any conditions that will cause harm to the patient and or caregiver.
- The health-care provider weighs the good versus the harm when considering wound treatments.
- The health-care provider puts the patient's interests foremost.

Remember

Doing good refers not only to the final outcome of a course of treatment but also to each individual treatment session. The health-care provider is expected to be able to acknowledge at the end of each treatment or encounter that more good than harm has been provided.

Nonmaleficence

The ethical principle of nonmaleficence refers to a professional obligation that all health-care providers owe to their patients. This is the obligation to cause or inflict no harm including deliberate harm, risk of harm, and harm that may occur during an act of doing good. Generally, health-care professionals discuss nonmaleficence in terms of not causing the death of a patient; however, it also means not causing pain or suffering, not causing incapacitation, not causing offense to others, and not depriving another person of a good life.

When considering nonmaleficence in wound management, the health-care provider considers the mental competency of the patient or designee when providing explanations

Remember

Inquire at the beginning, throughout, and at the end of each encounter what the patient has experienced. It is important to inform the patient and caregivers that wound care is not intended to cause pain. Therefore, ask each patient to inform the health-care provider throughout the encounter and at the end of each encounter of any discomfort or pain. If the patient reports discomfort or pain, adjust the treatment to reduce this to a level that is acceptable to each individual patient.

or information. It is also important to select treatments that cause little to no pain and to thoroughly discuss this with the patient or designee before pursuing any treatment or lack of treatment. Additionally, it is an important part of this ethical principle to be as culturally aware as possible while maintaining an open mind about the individual rationale for any action or reaction.

Fidelity

Within the field of health-care bioethics, the term fidelity is defined as promise-keeping.[1] In general, the individual who receives care from any health-care provider has an expectation that each health-care provider will keep any promises made directly to the patient, family, and or caregiver. Specifically, this means that when the health-care provider says he or she will do something, that is what is done, unless doing so is completely beyond the health-care provider's axis of control. In other words health-care providers do what they say they are going to do. For this reason, it is important that each health-care provider speak only for him or herself and his or her actions or expected actions. When providing wound care this means do not promise

Remember

Patients, family members, and caregivers may not hear all that is said by the health-care provider the first time it is said. Therefore, it is important to repeat information more than one time during an encounter. Have information such as wound care instructions, future appointments, and dietary recommendations written in the patient's spoken language and provided at each encounter. Ascertain the reading level of the patient, family, and caregivers before providing written materials. Pictures, if available may be more useful than written instructions.

or guarantee anything about the wound, the wound care, or future treatment that is not directly under one's control.

Role Fidelity

Role fidelity refers to the legal scope of practice of each health-care provider. Under specific levels of scope of practice, there are designated constraints. For example, a professional nurse cannot in most instances change an order for wound treatment without conferring directly with the prescribing health-care provider (MD, DPM, RNP, etc.). Promise-keeping relative to the health-care provider's role means faithfully practicing within the scope of that role. Additionally, it is important to recognize that wound care is not provided by one practitioner alone. Wound care is a team effort; each member of the team recognizes the benefits brought to the team by each team member. Within this team, each member must practice within the constraints of his or her scope of practice as well as within any constraints of the team.

Remember

A scope of practice is most often the result of traditions within a particular health-care specialty and legislation (state or national) that specifies the privileges of each health-care specialty. Each health-care provider who evaluates and/or provides wound care should have a thorough knowledge of his or her scope of practice and his or her role in the treatment of each patient who has a wound.

Veracity

According to the Oxford English Dictionary veracity is defined as "speaking or stating the truth; habitual observance of the truth; truthfulness."

In regards to patients with wounds, this truth or truthfulness connects the patient and the health-care provider. This connection means that it is expected that the patient tells the truth to the health-care provider and also that the health-care provider tells the truth to the patient or patient surrogate. In regards to wound care, this is not about some philosophical debate concerning what is really the truth; rather it is the disclosure of factual information from both parties. Traditionally, the fiduciary relationship that exists between health-care providers and the patients for whom they provide care is one of unique and special veracity. For example, the patient has the right to expect a higher level of veracity from his or her health-care provider than he or she may expect from others in general society. The health-care provider is bound by the concept of role fidelity as determined by his or her scope of practice.

In the past it was deemed acceptable for the health-care provider to tell the patient what he or she thought was best for the patient to know. In some fields this was known as benevolent deception. This form of paternalism was justified by saying that the individual patient could not understand or handle the truth about his or her condition, treatment, or prognosis. Unfortunately, this type of deception leads the health-care provider into what is commonly known in bioethics as a slippery slope argument.

Today, the health-care provider shares with the patient as much factual information as the health-care provider knows and that which the patient wants to know. This amount of truth is disclosed to assist the patient or surrogate in making well-informed, autonomous decisions.

Therapeutic Privilege

Therapeutic privilege refers to a legal exception under informed consent. Briefly, it means that the health-care provider does not obtain consent for care in situations such as a life-threatening emergency, patient incompetence, or patient mental instability. Exercising therapeutic privilege is best left to licensed physicians and is rare when providing care to patients with wounds.

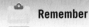

Remember

Provide truthful information within the scope of practice to patients and their surrogates.

Conflict of Interest

In general, the health-care professions are thought to exist primarily to render services to patients who need care. A conflict of interest arises when the health-care provider has or potentially has an interest in the patient other than the provider's obligation to protect and promote the patient's interests. The health-care provider should avoid these conflicts at all times. For example, there should be no financial incentive to evaluating or providing care to a patient with wounds. Such an example would include owning stock in the product or products that are recommended or prescribed for treatment. A conflict of interest would also exist if the health-care provider referred the patient to him or herself or to anyone with whom the provider has a financial or personal relationship. Practices such as providing bonuses at the end of the fiscal year may also be seen as a conflict of interest. Many health-care organizations have developed firm policies about what is determined

Remember

Examples of conflicts of interests occur when the health-care provider recommends that the patient purchases supplies from a medical supply company for which a referral bonus is received for patients referred to that vendor.

to be a conflict of interest; therefore, the health-care provider needs to keep him- or herself updated continually regarding these policies.

Confidentiality

In respect to health care, confidentiality refers to the necessity that each health-care provider hold in strict confidence information that is discovered about the patient during the course of the health-care practice. Generally, the patient has the right to expect that any knowledge of his or her condition be discussed or made available only to those health-care providers who will need such information for care provision or reimbursement purposes. The patient also has the right to expect that he or she selects what health-care information and to whom that health-care information may be released.

In some areas, under legislation, the patient's rights are superceded by the need to provide safety to the public. One example is the requirement in many geographic locations to inform a public health entity of communicable diseases. In most cases such an example is uncommon in wound care.

 Remember

It is the responsibility of each health-care provider to be aware of current organizational policies or legislation concerning confidentiality.

Justice

Aside from autonomy, there is no bioethical concept quite as controversial as justice. Originally, justice was a philosophical concept that has been debated over the centuries. However, the health-care provider confronted with a patient who needs wound evaluation and care, does not want to be debating an esoteric concept. Therefore in the field of wound care, the most common type of justice that is encountered, is that of distributive justice. The various theories of distributive justice strive to connect specific elements of the patient with distributions of benefits and burdens that can be justified at that specific time and place.

Distributive justice seems to imply a fair and equal distribution of health-care resources; however, this would also imply that there were enough resources available at any given time for all who might require them. Obviously, this is not the current situation found in the world at this time. Therefore, it becomes the responsibility of each health-care provider to treat each patient as equitably as possible within the organizational structure and available resources. When this does not seem

Remember

An ethical dilemma occurs when one is confronted with a wound that has been vigorously treated, but does not respond to a variety of treatments. The wound may not heal at any time in the foreseeable future therefore continuing to consume resources that may not be plentiful. Include the entire wound team in discussions of such situations and develop appropriate plans of care that include counseling for the patient, family, and caregivers. These team members must assist all other involved health-care providers to critically evaluate:

1. What specifically can be done to resolve the wound?

2. What must be done to resolve the wound?

3. What must not be done to resolve the wound?

4. In what time frame and what manner should the wound be resolved?

likely, the health-care provider should ask for an ethics committee consultation or consult directly with an ethicist or a more senior health-care provider.

In summary, a variety of bioethical concepts have been defined and discussed relevant to providing evaluation and care to individuals with wounds. It is important that all health-care providers remain ever vigilant in recognizing situations and applying these concepts.

INTERNET RESOURCES

The following Internet resources provide a variety of materials to assist with ethics and ethical decision making:

- **The University of Pennsylvania bioethics site**

  —http://www.bioethics.upenn.edu/

- **The President's Council on Bioethics (USA)**

  —http://www.bioethics.net/

- **The National Center for Ethics of the Veterans Health Administration**

  —http://bioethics.gov/ http://www.va.gov/ethics/

- **The Nuffield Council on Bioethics**

  —http://www.nuffieldbioethics.org/

- **National Reference Center for Bioethics Literature, the Kennedy Institute of Ethics**

  —http://www.georgetown.edu/research/nrcbl/

- **American Medical Association bioethics site**

  —http://www.ama-assn.org/ama/pub/category/2416.html

- **University of San Diego site has comprehensive information on ethical theory and applied ethics**

  —http://ethics.acusd.edu/index.asp

- **National Institute of Health**

  —http://www.bioethics.nih.gov/resources/index.html

- **The Hastings Center**
  —http://www.thehastingscenter.org/
- **The Center for Health Ethics and Law at the West Virginia University Health ethical issues for professionals and non-professionals**
  —www.hsc.wvu.edu/chel
- **Cardiff Centre for Ethics Law and Society (UK)**
  —http://www.ccels.cardiff.ac.uk/literature/issue/index.html
- **University of Minnesota Center for Bioethics**
  —http://www.bioethics.umn.edu/
- **American Nurses Association Center for Ethics and Human Rights**
  —http://www.nursingworld.org/ethics/

REFERENCES

1. Beauchamp TL, Childress J F. *Principles of Biomedical Ethics.* New York, NY: Oxford University Press; 2001.
2. Edge RS, Groves JR. *Ethics of Health Care: A Guide for Clinical Practice.* 3rd ed. Clifton Park, NY: Thomson Delmar Learning; 2006.

SUGGESTED READING

American Nurses Association. *Code of Ethics for Nurses with Interpretive Statements.* Washington, DC: Author; 2001.

American Nurses Association. *Nursing's Social Policy Statement.* 2nd ed. Washington, DC: Author; 2003.

Angelucci PA. Ethics in practice. Grasping the concept of medical futility. *Nursing Management.* 2006; 37(2):12–14.

Austin W. Nursing ethics in an era of globalization. *Advances in Nursing Science.* 2001;24(2):1–18.

The Belmont Report: Ethical Principles and Guidelines for the protection of human subjects of research. Available at: http://ohsr.od. nih.gov/guidelines/Belmont.html. Accessed January 02, 2006.

At least 25% of older adults will be uninsured at some point during the years preceding eligibility for Medicare. *Nursing Economics*. May/June 2006; 24(3):165 (journal article - brief item).

Breier-Mackie S. Patient autonomy and medical paternity: can nurses help doctors listen to patients? *Nursing Ethic*. 2001;8(6):510–521.

Butts J, Rich K. *Nursing Ethics: Across the Curriculum and Into Practice*. Boston, MA: Jones & Bartlett; 2005.

Chandra A, Willis W, Miller K. (2005). Patient-physician relationships in the managed care environment—a comparative analysis of various models. *Hospital Topics*. 2005;83(2): 36–39.

Cherry B, Jacob S. *Contemporary Nursing: Issues, Trends, and Management*. 3rd ed. Philadelphia, PA: Mosby; 2005.

Davis AJ. Global influence of American nursing: some ethical issues. *Nursing Ethics*. 1999;6(2):118–125.

Eldh A, Ekman I, Ehnfors M. Conditions for patient participation and non-participation in health care. *Nursing Ethics*. 2006;13(5): 503–514.

Erlen JA. When patients and families disagree. *Orthopaedic Nursing*. 2005;24(4): 279–282.

Fleck LM. The costs of caring: Who pays? Who profits? Who panders? *Hastings Center Report*. May–June 2006: 13–16.

Gruskin S. Human rights and ethics in public health. *American Journal of Public Health*. 2006;96(11): 1903–1905.

Hanssen I. An intercultural nursing perspective on autonomy. *Nursing Ethics*. 2004;11(1):28–41.

Harper MG. Ethical multiculturalism: an evolutionary concept analysis. *Advances in Nursing Science*. 2006;29(2): 110–124.

Hickman SE, Hammes BJ, Moss H, Tolle SW. Hope for the future: achieving the original intent of advance directives. *Hastings Center Report*. 2005;35(6):S26–S30.

Hyland D. An exploration of the relationship between patient autonomy and patient advocacy: implications for nursing practice. *Nursing Ethics*. 2002;9(5):472–482.

Izumi S. Bridging western ethics and Japanese local ethics by listening to nurses' concerns. *Nursing Ethics*. 2006);13(3): 275–283.

Jacobs BB, Taylor C. Medical futility in the natural attitude. *Advances in Nursing Science*. 2005;28(4):288–305.

Jonsdottir H, Litchfield M, Pharris MD. The relational core of nursing practice as partnership. *Journal of Advanced Nursing*. 2004;47(3):241–250.

Loewy EH, Loewy RS. *Changing health care systems from ethical, economic, and cross-cultural perspectives*. New York, NY: Kluwer Academic; 2002.

Loewy EH, Loewy RS. *The ethics of terminal care: orchestrating the end of life*. New York, NY: Kluwer Academic; 2002.

McCabe C. Nurse-patient communication: an exploration of patient's experiences. *Journal of Clinical Nursing*. 2004;13: 41–49.

Monson MS. What to know about duty to report. *Nursing Management*. 2005;36(5):14–16, 65.

Pelton LH. Getting what we deserve. *Humanist*. 2006;66(4): 14–17.

Peternelj-Taylor CA, Yonge O. Exploring boundaries in the Nurse-Client relationship: professional roles and responsibilities. *Perspectives in Psychiatric Care*. 2003;39(2):55–66.

Sire JW. *The Universe Next Door: A Basic Worldview Catalogue*. Downer's Grove, IL: InterVarsity Press ; 2004.

Starrs JM. The medical futility debate: treatment at any cost? *Journal of Gerontological Nursing*. 2006;32(5):13–16.

Tarlier DS. Beyond caring: the moral and ethical bases of responsive nurse-patient relationships. *Nursing Philosophy*. 2004;5(3): 230–241.

Treadwell K, Cram N. Managed healthcare and federal health programs. *Journal of Clinical Engineering*. Jan/Mar 2004; 36–42.

Tsai F-C D. Eye on religion: Confucianism, autonomy, and patient care. *Southern Medical Journal*. June 2006;99(6): 685–687.

United Nations: Universal Declaration of Human Rights. Available at: http://www.un.org/Overviewrights.hml. Accessed January 02, 2006 January:

Von Bruck M. An ethics of justice in a cross-cultural context. *Buddhist-Christian Studies*. 2006;26:61–77.

Woods DJ. Forty million uninsured: the ethics of public policy. *Public Integrity*. 2006;8(2):149–164.

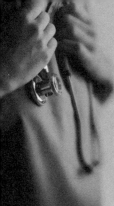

Chapter 2

PRINCIPLES OF SKIN AND WOUND CARE

KEY POINTS

- Suggested bathing, soaps, and general skin care.
- Acne treatment rationale and common actions of over the counter (OTC) and prescription therapies.
- Concepts for use in sun protection of the skin.
- Nutrition effective for skin care.
- Commonly used lotions and creams including rationale for use.
- Definitions and concepts of wound healing, repair, and types of wounds.

DAILY SKIN CARE

Following are effective measures to take for care of the skin of both men and women on a daily basis.

- Bathing
  - Avoid excessive washing; daily washing may not be necessary
  - Use tepid water avoiding temperature extremes, especially hot water
  - Avoid overaggressive use of washcloths that may exfoliate and remove stratum corneum
  - Use a gentle, nondrying bar or liquid soap
    - Each individual should have his or her own soap, no sharing of soap products
    - Antibacterial soap is not necessary unless prescribed
    - Moisturizing soaps such as Dove, Keri, Cetaphil, and Basis are best
    - Pure Ivory Soap can be very drying and irritating
    - Axilla, groin, and perianal area may require soap; not every body part requires soap
  - Gently pat dry the skin and avoid abrasives and rubbing
  - Apply a water-based lotion twice a day directly onto damp skin and allow to air dry
  - Exfoliants like a loofah are not necessary unless prescribed

— Use a gentle adult shampoo once every 7 days unless otherwise indicated

- Children's shampoo is not effective for adults
- Avoid hair products with alcohol, lead, and other toxins

• Acne skin care

— Acne is a disease of pilosebaceous units in the skin. The sebaceous glands secrete sebum—an oily substance—through the opening at the follicles (Figure 2-1). The most common locations for acne outbreaks are the face, upper chest, and back, due to the dense population of pilosebaceous units in these areas. Secreted sebum, the hair, and keratinocytes in these pilosebaceous units form a plug, which prohibits the sebum from reaching the skin's surface.

- Skin bacteria attract white blood cells resulting in inflammation and the formation of a pimple.
- These enlarged follicles, once plugged, form the acne comedo or lesion. A white lesion is a closed comedo while one that reaches the surface of the skin is an open comedo. These surface lesions turn black as the sebum is exposed to air.

  ○ Some acne patients also experience papule($\leq$ 5 mm), pustules (dome-shaped), macules (flat, temporary, red spot after acne lesion is healed), nodules (often painful, dome- or irregularly-shaped, solid), or cysts (sac-like and larger than pustules, often very painful and may result in significant scarring).[2]

- Acne contributors include[1]

  ○ Fluctuating hormones
  ○ Family history
  ○ Medications

  - Anticonvulsants (phenytoin sodium, valproic acid)
  - Antiinflammatory corticosteroids (prednisone)
  - Immunosuppressants (azathioprine)
  - Those medications used to stimulate the thyroid gland

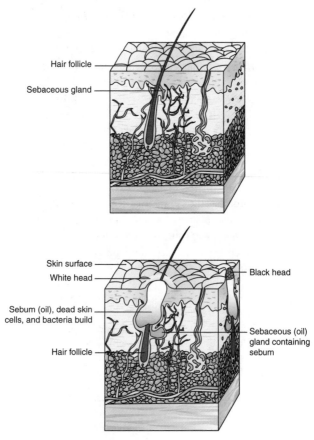

Figure 2–1 Sebaceous follicle. A, normal. B, plugged with acne.

- Pressure on skin from athletic equipment and tight clothing
- Greasy cosmetics
- Grease in the environment (e.g., working as a cook or machinist)

- Irritants in the environment (e.g., increased humidity or air pollution)
- Stress may exacerbate flairs
- Hard scrubbing causes skin irritation that may trigger inflammation
- Squeezing or picking at the lesions may cause bacteria to be pushed away from the surface and into the pilosebaceous units creating comedo formation
- Over-the-counter and prescription acne medications (Table 2–1)

— Each client who has acne should be encouraged to find the soap or cleanser that assists him or her in management of this condition. In some clients the mildest soap is the most effective.

- Remember acne is not caused by dirt.
- Diet does not play a significant role in most adolescent cases of acne, but if a particular food seems to have an apparent relationship to a flair, it is best to moderate intake of that food or fluid.
- Acne treatment is a process that often takes up to 8 weeks before therapeutic benefits are observable; therefore, the treatment should not be stopped precipitously.

- Sun protection
  — Use sunscreen daily on all areas exposed to the sun
  — Apply 20 minutes to 1 hour before sun exposure and reapply liberally and often
  — Use an appropriate sunscreen for skin type and activity
  — Use sunscreen with UVA and UVB protection
  — Avoid sun exposure from 10 AM to 2 PM
  — Wear tightly woven clothing
  — Wear a hat with a wide brim. Note: Baseball caps do not protect the ears and neck

Table 2–1 Common Acne Treatments

Ingredient	Action
Allantoin	Stimulates healthy tissue
Antibiotics (various topical and systemic)	Controls bacteria and reduces inflammation
Azelaic acid	Creates normal skin
Benzyl peroxide	Kills acne bacteria
Glycolic acid	Renews skin
Green tea	Regulates sebum; decreases amount at skin level
Licorice root	Evens skin tone
Olive leaf	Kills acne bacteria
Oral contraceptives	Used in females to reduce ovarian and adrenal production of androgens
Retinoids	Unplug comedones and decrease new comedone formation; reduce size of sebaceous glands and decrease sebum production
Salicylic acid	Unclogs skin pores; effective in reducing severity & duration of outbreaks. Skin sheds more evenly.
Sulfur	Dries sebum; has antibacterial effect
Tea tree oil	Reduces inflammation; especially in oily skin

From Acne review chart. Available at: www.acne-review.com/images/acne-chart-2-gif. Accessed January 25, 2008.

— Avoid tanning salons
— Review medications with a pharmacist before sun activity
— Remember that high altitudes intensify sun exposure
— Perform an overall skin inspection daily

- Nutrition
  - Eat a balanced diet
  - Drink enough noncaffeinated fluids throughout the day; 2 to 2 1/2 quarts a day (check with health-care provider if on fluid restriction)
  - Remember that high altitudes can cause dehydration; be sure to increase fluids
  - Avoid using tobacco products
- Skin lotions and creams
  - Skin lotions and creams are used to restore water and lipids to the epidermis, especially to dry skin
  - Dry skin is an inherited trait common in atopic patients with a personal or family history of
    - Hay fever
    - Asthma
    - Dry skin
    - Eczema
  - More common in winter months or whenever environmental humidity is low (e.g., air-conditioned buildings)
  - Dry skin most commonly occurs on the hands and lower legs
  - The initial appearance of dry skin is rough texture followed by fine white lines and scales that becomes thicker tan or brown scales or sheets.
  - The differences between creams and lotions are:
    - Creams are thicker than lotion
    - Creams are more lubricating than lotions
    - Some creams may contain less water than the lotion of the same name/brand
  - Brands of lighter creams:
    - Cetaphil cream
    - DML cream
    - Moisturel cream
    - Nutraplus cream

— Brands of lighter lotions:
  - Cetaphil lotion
  - DML lotion
  - Nutraderm lotion
  - Moisturel lotion
  - Eucerin lotion
  - Keri lotion

— Special preparations:
  - Sarna lotion
    ◦ Contains menthol and camphor
    ◦ Controls pruritus
  - Lac-Hydrin
    ◦ Contains ammonium lactate
    ◦ Highly effective in treating very dry skin
    ◦ Very expensive
    ◦ Available by prescription only
  - Amlactin
    ◦ Similar to Lac-Hydrin
    ◦ Less expensive
    ◦ Available without prescription
  - Alpha hydroxyl acid moisturizers
    ◦ May be slightly more effective than other creams
    ◦ More expensive
    ◦ May not be worth the extra cost according to some skin experts
  - Thicker creams and ointments are
    ◦ Greasy
    ◦ Substantial
    ◦ Long lasting
  - Applied in the evening or at bedtime due to their weight and greasiness

— Brands of thicker creams and ointments:
- Vaseline petroleum jelly
- Aquaphor
- Eucerin cream
- Solid cooking fat (e.g., Crisco)

• Application of creams and lotions
  — Apply lubricants after washing when the skin has just been hydrated
  — Pat skin dry and apply lotion or cream (some experts disagree that lubricants may be applied to wet skin)
  — Apply lubricants as frequently as necessary to keep skin soft
  — Some lubricants contain dimethecone—a water repellant—which may require less frequent application
  — Most moisturizers may be used on any part of the body (face, body, eyelids, and hands) unless otherwise specified
  — Check with health-care provider regarding which brands to purchase rather than spending large sums of money on cosmetic company brands

DEFINITIONS AND CONCEPTS OF WOUND HEALING AND REPAIR

An understanding of basic definitions as they apply to wound care is necessary in order to grasp the concepts and principles of wound healing and repair.

Definitions and Concepts

• Wound: disruption of normal integumentary anatomic structure and function.
• Wound healing: complex sequence of events initiated when an injury occurs and ends when complete wound closure and successful, functional scar tissue has organized (up to 18 months after wound closure).

- Acute wound: disruption in normal integumentary anatomic structure and function; commonly caused by trauma or surgery; healing occurs in an expected amount of time without complications.
  — "A disruption in the integrity of the skin and underlying tissues that progress through the healing process in a timely and uncomplicated manner."[3]
- Chronic wound: disruption in normal integumentary anatomic structure and function commonly caused by pressure, diabetes mellitus, diminished circulation, inadequate nutritional status, immunodeficiencies, infection, or some other causes; healing may occur in an extended amount of time with complications.
  — NOTE: *not all chronic wounds heal.*
  — NOTE: Medicare considers wounds that are 30 days old or more to be chronic wounds.
  — Includes wounds that "fail to progress through a normal, orderly, and timely sequence of repair or wounds that pass through the repair process without restoring anatomic and functional results."[4]
- Recalcitrant wound: disruption in normal integumentary anatomic structure and function; healing is stubborn, defiant, refractory, or unmanageable.
  — NOTE: also known as difficult-to-heal wounds.
- Stunned wound: disruption in normal integumentary anatomic structure and function, which initially begins on an expected healing trajectory and then plateaus and/or becomes recalcitrant; may also be called "stalled wound."
- Partial thickness wound: disruption in normal integumentary anatomic structure and function through the epidermis, extending into but not through the dermis.
- Full thickness wound: disruption in normal integumentary anatomic structure and function extending through the dermis involving subcutaneous tissue, which may include muscle and/or bone.

Wound Healing and Repair

- The determination of the wound healing phase describes the biological phase of tissue repair as observed by the provider and has clinical value in determining the goal and type of treatment as well as financial reimbursement for wound treatment.

  — Acute phase indicates an orderly progression through the phases of wound healing (inflammation, proliferation, epithelialization, and remodeling). This is observed in acute wounds.

  — Chronic phase indicates that the orderly progression is not occurring and the wound is chronic in nature.

  — Absent phase indicates that the wound has not progressed through a specific healing phase.

- Hemostasis: injury causes tissue disruption and hemorrhage follows filling the wound and exposing blood to extracellular matrix components (ECM). A clot forms as a result of platelet aggregation and degranulation which activates factor XII (Hageman factor) causing hemostasis. During coagulation, a fibrinous clot forms filling the wound space. As fibrinolysis begins, the clot dissolves and cells migrate into the wound space allowing the next stage of healing to proceed.

- Acute inflammation: normal and first phase of healing lasting 3 to 4 days from the initial wounding. As the fibrin clot dissolves, dilating capillaries become more permeable allowing fluid into the injury site which activates the complement system. This system is a series of interacting, soluble proteins that induce lysis and destruction of target cells. It also helps bind neutrophils to bacteria thereby facilitating phagocytosis. The peak number of neutrophils appear in the wound within 24 to 48 hours after injury and their numbers decrease after 3 days if no infection is present. Two to three days after injury tissue macrophages arrive and are followed by lymphocytes. The macrophages are an important source of biological regulators (i.e., cytokines, growth factors, bioactive lipid products, and proteolytic enzymes). All of these are essential for normal healing. This phase may not be observed by the home-care provider due to the timing of wound development.

- Absence of inflammation: this represents the body's inability to present an immune response and may be present in individuals with immune compromise, diabetes, overuse of antiseptics, drug or radiation therapy, or severe ischemia.
- Chronic inflammation: persists for weeks to months and is generally caused by prolonged trauma to the wounded area. This occurs when macrophages and neutrophils are not phagocytosing necrotic tissue, ingesting foreign debris, or fighting infection. This is also a result of histamine release from mast cells and reflex hyperemia caused by vasodilatation in the surrounding vessels.
- Acute proliferation: normal and second phase of healing; begins 3 to 4 days post wounding and may last 4 to 24 days in acute wounds.
- Chronic proliferation: often occurs when an infection is present in the wound impairing the proliferation process. The wound is "stuck" and not progressing to the next phase. May last up to 11 months in chronic wounds.
- Acute epithelialization: this begins concurrently with hemostasis and begins a few hours after wounding. It will also overlap in other phases and is a normal part of wound healing.
- Chronic epithelialization: cells stack up on each other and present as a ridge along the edge of the wound that is rolled, thickened, and fibrotic. Hyperkeratosis is one abnormality of epithelialization and represents an overgrowth of the horny layer.
- Absence of epithelialization: may be due to intrinsic, extrinsic, or iatrogenic causes.
- Acute remodeling: last and longest phase of healing; collagen is remodeling and scar formation is occurring. Elevated collagenolytic activity has been detected at 20 years after wounding. Generally, the wound will attain an 80% tensile strength; 2 years is a common time frame.
- Chronic remodeling: formation of keloid scarring.

- Absence of remodeling: may be due to intrinsic, extrinsic, or iatrogenic causes and is represented by a wound that does not scar to closure.

Superficial Wound Healing

- Superficial wound healing includes first-degree burns, contusions, and stage I pressure ulcers, which are usually caused by friction and/or shear or a combination of friction and shear.
- This type of skin damage may be the first indication of deeper tissue wounding or trauma.
- The healing process stimulates the inflammatory process of repair that may begin within hours of the damage.
- The involved soft tissues heal themselves with time. The goal of any provider intervention at this point is to restore functional activities as quickly as possible such as treatment of athletes to reduce pain and loss of athletic activity time.

Primary Intention and Delayed Primary Wound Healing

- Primary intention healing: wound edges are brought together for closure. The following is necessary for primary intention healing to occur:
  - No major loss of subcutaneous tissue
  - Wound edges are smooth and clean cut
  - Wound is not contaminated with microorganisms or foreign bodies
  - Wound edges must be brought together without tension.
- This type of healing occurs rapidly and is less visible than partial thickness healing or secondary intention healing. Epithelial cells migrate rapidly—cells may migrate from sebaceous or sweat glands and hair follicles creating islands of epithelial tissue and more rapid healing—and the migration may be complete within 72 hours of primary closure.
- When primary intention healing is effective it leaves minimal residual scarring and attains closure in 3 to 18 days. Sutures

or staples may be removed (if no untoward signs or symptoms are present) in approximately

— Face: 4 to 6 days

— Neck: 6 to 10 days

— Back: 10 to 14 days

— Abdomen: 7 to 10 days

— Extremities: 10 to 18 days

* Skin edges may also be brought together and glued for primary intention closure.

* Delayed primary healing: occurs when wounds are contaminated with foreign bodies or microorganisms; have a large loss of tissue; closure by primary intention creates intolerable tension on the tissues; the patient is placed at risk for infection if the wound is closed by primary intention.

— In delayed primary healing, the wound is left open with a dressing in place and sutures are usually placed in the subcutaneous tissue and the fascia. The closure occurs in 5 to 7 days or after the risk of infection is significantly reduced and/or the loss of tissue has been replaced.

Partial Thickness Wound Healing

* Partial thickness wounds heal by repair. Repair is the resurfacing of the wound with new epidermal cells and begins immediately after injury. Inflammation is initiated and epidermal cells at the wound edges and from the dermal appendages (sweat glands, hair follicles, and sebaceous glands) migrate to the wound to assist with the resurfacing.

* When dermal appendages (hair follicles, sebaceous, or sweat glands) are present, epidermal cells may appear as island-like areas on the wound surface. These increase the resurfacing rate and most often the newly resurfaced area cannot be distinguished from the surrounding noninjured tissue.

Secondary Intention Wound Healing

* Secondary intention wound healing is chosen for wounds with full thickness skin loss; when the wound has disconti-

nuity or gaps; when the wound has irregular edges that cannot be adequately approximated; when the wound edges or margins are nonviable; when the wound has significant amounts of foreign debris and/or high number or microorganisms; and when the wound has skin necrosis.

- Wounds that heal by secondary intention are left open with a dressing to close by contraction or secondary intention. This occurs as the myofibroblasts draw the wound edges together.

- Wounds that heal by secondary intention heal by regeneration not repair. There is relatively little epithelialization. Scar tissue is formed. This scar tissue does not replicate the tissue it is replacing and the surface tissue will not equal the tensile strength or elasticity of the original tissue. The scar width (if the patient does not form keloids) will be approximately 10% of the original defect.[6]

- Secondary intention wound healing also occurs when there is a defect that is too small to close by primary intention. Additionally, split-thickness grafts cover some wounds especially if the wound is in an area where contraction will cause disfigurement or nonfunctional deformities.

Acute Wound Healing

- Acute wound healing has been referred to as a cascade of overlapping events that are expected to occur in a predictable manner. This cascade presents as a series of 4 phases.

  — Phase 1, Hemostasis: tissue has been injured and hemorrhage has occurred. This proceeds through a cascade of platelet activation and degradation to activation of the complement cascade, which results in blood clotting and hemostasis allowing the next phase of healing to proceed.

  — Phase 2, Inflammation: acute inflammation is initiated with the injury and lasts 3 to 7 days. This phase establishes the biologic cascade of overall wound healing. The most often observed signs and symptoms are

    ▪ change in color of the surrounding skin—red, blue, or purple

- increase in temperature of the wounded area
- edema and/or swelling in the area of the wound
- induration in the area
- sensation loss or increase, or itching, or pain in area
- loss of function (dependent on location)
  - The injury to the tissue initiates hemostasis with activation of clotting factors which are responding to the collagen and microfibrils released from the subendothelial layers exposed by the injury (in the case of open acute wounds). This develops a fibrin clot which initially closes the wound and prevents further blood and body fluid loss. It is at this time that the platelets release platelet-derived growth factor, epidermal growth factor, and chemoattractants. These substances stimulate mast cells to release histamine—a vasoactive component—and also stimulate the migration of granulocytes and macrophages to the area. The histamine causes the surrounding vessels to dilate and increase their permeability. This creates vasocongestion and serous fluid leakage into the wound bed resulting in the wound becoming erythematous, edematous, warm, and exudative. Histamine also stimulates the migration of endothelial cells and attracts leukocytic cells to the wound.
  - Platelets produce chemoattractants, which activate clotting factors. Fibrin breakdown attracts leukocytes to the wound bed (one of the most powerful chemoattractants is transforming growth factor-beta, while some others are bacterial products). The first to arrive, usually within 6 hours, are the polymorphonuclear leukocytes (PMNs). These white blood cells provide initial protection from bacterial invasion. One type of PMN that arrives within the first 24 hours is the neutrophil, which remains from 6 hours to several days. These cells are granulocytic and phagocytic in a hypoxic acidotic environment (created by hemostasis).

These cells produce a superoxide that fights bacteria and enhances the effect of antibiotics. If the bacterial count is high, so is the neutrophil count and the amount of time the neutrophils stay in the wound will be prolonged. The neutrophil is the primary cell responsible for cleansing the wound of microorganisms and a lack of significant numbers of neutrophils will retard wound healing. In approximately 4 days after the injury, macrophages arrive and gradually replace the PMNs. These cells function in a low-oxygen, high-acidotic environment to phagocytize debris and control infection by microorganism ingestion and excretion of ascorbic acid, hydrogen peroxide, and lactic acid. It is the macrophage (derived from the monocyte) that assumes the "director" role from this point forward in the wound healing process. Macrophages secrete angiogenesis growth factor (AGF), which stimulates the budding of endothelial cells for initiation of neoangiogenesis (new blood vessel formation). Additionally, the macrophages control various processes in wound healing and convert macromolecules into amino acids and sugars needed for healing. They also secrete lactate to stimulate collagen synthesis.

- Macrophages in combination with dead platelets produce fibroblast-stimulating factor which signals the fibroblasts to migrate during the last stage of the inflammatory phase. Fibroblasts are the cells that build the matrix of collagen during the proliferative phase. At this phase they begin to differentiate and some become myofibroblasts during the later stage of inflammation. The myofibroblasts have the ability to expand and contract thereby drawing the wound together and influencing the rate and amount of wound contraction.
- The macrophage is thought to live months to years and remains in the wound fluid during all phases of healing.

- ○ If the wound is necrotic or infected, the inflammation phase is prolonged and the healing process is delayed.
- ○ If the wound is partial thickness, the epithelial cells begin resurfacing immediately. The epithelial cells also debride partial thickness wounds through release of lytic enzymes. Migration of these cells is dependent on oxygen. Debridement cannot occur if the oxygen level is low.

— Phase 3, Proliferation: components of this phase are granulation and epithelialization and are part of full thickness healing. If the wound is healing by secondary intention contraction will also occur. There are overlapping characteristics of this phase:

- Fibroplasia: development of collagen matrix also known as granulation.
- Wound contraction: the drawing together of the wound edges.
- Initial granulation tissue looks like pale pink buds becoming more beefy and bright red as the tissue fills with new blood vessels (neoangiogenesis). The collagen matrix is filled with a thick capillary bed that supplies the nutrients and oxygen necessary for healing.
- This initial granulation tissue is not a replication of the tissue it is replacing.
- During proliferation, the vascular response initiated in inflammation must sustain the perfusion of nutrients and oxygen to support the fibroblasts, myofibroblasts, endothelial cells, and epidermal cells (cells of repair).
- The macrophages and neutrophils work to control infection as long as the wound is open. For the combination of these activities to continue, the wound must be kept warm as this stimulates cellular division. It is also necessary for the wound to remain moist during this stage as the moisture contains ions that attract the necessary cells.

- The responder cells, fibroblasts, myofibroblasts, endothelial cells, and epidermal cells are highly active during proliferation. The fibroblasts extrude collagen chains which aggregate into procollagen (a triple helix). The procollagen cleaves becoming tropocollagen molecules. These molecules associate with other like molecules forming a collagen fibril which then produces disorganized filaments. Intermolecular cross-linkage is the organization and bonding of the filaments.

- Fibroplasia is the official name for this process of the cross-linkage forming the collagen matrix for wound tensile strength and durability. A high degree of organization and cross-linkage results in a higher tensile strength or a stronger remodeling of the scar tissue. Frequent disruption of the healing may create more disorganization resulting in longer or no healing as well as larger, less elastic scarification.

- Another connective tissue synthesized by the fibroblast is elastin, so named because of its elasticity. Its major function is to maintain tissue shape and it is found in the urinary bladder, lungs, blood vessels, and skin. Glycoproteins, laminin, and fibronectin, are fiber-forming molecules that work together with elastin to provide structural and metabolic support to other tissues.

- The collagen matrix is composed of elastin plus the new vascular network and visually looks like a red granule piled on top of other red granules, hence the name "granulation tissue."

- Wound contraction is then initiated by the myofibroblasts. These cells connect themselves to the margins of the wound and exert an inward pulling force on the epidermal layer. A ring of myofibroblasts is created and is similar to a picture frame that is beneath the skin contracting the wound. In the beginning, these contractile forces are equal; however, the shape of the ring is a predictor of how rapidly the wound will heal.

- Linear wounds contract rapidly. For example, surgical wounds have minimal contraction response.
- Square or rectangular wounds contract at a moderate pace.
- Circular wounds contract slowly.
- It is important to control the wound contraction in all wounds but especially in specific areas such as the hand, neck, or face. Uncontrolled, rapid contraction may cause disfigurement and excessive scarring.
- NOTE: abnormalities in the healing at this stage may result in serious medical problems. During the first 3 weeks postoperatively, the average patient is at highest risk for wound dehiscence, opening of wound edges in a previously closed wound healed by primary intention, or wound evisceration (a medical emergency).

- Epithelialization: Within a few hours of the injury the body begins reepithelialization. Cells that are normally firmly attached to the underlying dermis and marginal basal cells change cellular adhesion properties, begin to lose their firm adhesion, and migrate in a leapfrog or train-like fashion across the provisional matrix. When cells meet horizontally the movement is stopped. This is called contact inhibition. If the wound is a surgical sutured one, the epidermal migration is initiated within 24 hours and is usually completed within 48 to 72 hours postoperatively in healthy adults.

- Other wound types often result in trauma to the skin including tissue degeneration with broad, indistinct, and difficult to visualize edges. These wounds often form a thickening, rolling inward epidermis. If trauma is repetitive, the wound edges become indurated, firm, fibrotic, and scarred.

- When the resurfacing has occurred, the epithelial cells differentiate and mature into type I collagen. The new skin has approximately a 15% tensile strength at this point and must be treated carefully including avoidance of trauma.

— Phase 4, Maturation or Remodeling: collagen synthesis and collagen lysis requires a balance in this stage. Collagenase, an enzyme, is produced during inflammation, continues in proliferation, and is the regulator of fibroplasia and the synthesis/lysis process.

  ▪ Maturing wounds have an increase in collagen lysis and this process is not oxygen dependent. Synthesis is oxygen dependent and too much oxygen may be the cause of hypertrophy in the granulation tissue. It is also known that some individuals have a genetic inhibition of lysis; this will create an imbalance in synthesis and lysis.

  ▪ Scar formation continues during this stage with fibronectin being laid down and the accumulation of large bundles of type I collagen. A new scar will have a red or rosy appearance due to small vessels which gradually retract. If the scar is red or rosy in color, remodeling is still in progress. The entire process takes from 3 weeks to 2 years postinjury.

Chronic Wound Healing

• Chronic wounds deviate from an expected sequence of repair. This deviance may be in terms of time, appearance, or response to treatment. They become "stuck" or "stalled" and do not progress through the phases of healing in a predictable, organized manner without intervention.

• It is important to identify the factors that contribute to wound chronicity as early as possible to improve the prognosis and outcomes as well as to reduce the costs and variability of care.

• The following factors affect wound healing:

  — Iatrogenic factors: factors related to the way the wound is managed

    ▪ Inappropriate wound care/treatment
    ▪ Inattention to contributing pathology
    ▪ Local ischemia
    ▪ Pressure

- Trauma
- Patient/caregiver nonadherence
— Extrinsic factors: related to sources in the environment that affect the body or the wound
  - Irradiation
  - Medication
  - Psychological or physiological stress
  - Wound bioburden, necrotic tissue, and infection
  - Other therapies that impair healing
— Intrinsic factors: related to medical status or physiologic properties within the patient
  - Age
  - Chronic diseases
  - Immunosuppression
  - Neuropathy
  - Malnutrition
— Nutrition and hydration: assessment and reassessment on a planned basis
  - Nutritional problems with wounds: direct and indirect
  - CBC, transferrin, prealbumin, albumin, zinc, 72-hour food and fluid log, current and recent weights including weight changes
  - High risk for malnutrition
  - Malnutrition red flags
- Protein needs in the normal healthy adult (nonpregnant, nonathlete) are 0.8/kg/day, or 58 to 63 g for males and 46 to 50 g for females.
- Determine weight in kg by taking weight in lbs divided by 2.2. For example, 140 kg ÷ 2.2 lbs = 63.5 kg
- Multiply the kg weight by 0.8 g/kg. This determines the recommended daily allowance (RDA) for protein.

  For example, 63.5 kg × 0.8 g/kg = 50.8 g protein RDA per day

- NOTE: the patient with a wound may require additional protein for wound repair and healing. Consider a referral to the dietitian (RD).
- Function of protein
  — wound repair
  — clotting factor production
  — white blood cell production and migration
  — cell-mediated phagocytosis
  — fibroblast proliferation
  — neovascularization
  — collagen synthesis
  — epithelial cell proliferation
  — wound remodeling
- Protein deficiency results in
  — impaired healing
  — edema
  — lymphopenia
  — impaired cellular immunity
- Be sure to verify the patient's laboratory tests with the specific laboratory used because each laboratory has their own established normal levels. Therefore, it is these levels that should be used in the evaluation of each client's results.

  NOTE: laboratory values are most useful as a tool to assess long-term nutrition changes because normal values may still be found in the patient who is malnourished.

  — Serum Albumin: normal 3.5–5.0 g/dL
    - 2.8–3.5 g/dL for nutritional analysis indicates compromised protein status
    - ↓2.8 g/dL indicates possible kwashiorkor—malnutrition caused by lack of protein while consuming adequate energy
    - Causes of abnormally low albumin levels:
      ○ Infection

- Poor protein intake
- Burns
- Trauma
- Congestive heart failure
- Fluid overload
- Severe hepatic insufficiency
- Function of albumin:
  - Visceral protein
  - Controls osmotic equilibrium
  - Albumin deficiency causes generalized edema, which slows oxygen diffusion and metabolic transport mechanisms from capillaries to cell membranes.

— Prealbumin: normal 20–50 mg/dL (also known as thyroxine-binding prealbumin)
  - Be sure to verify with each laboratory!
  - NOTE: useful in monitoring short-term changes in visceral protein due to its half-life of 2 days. Reflects what the patient ingests, absorbs, digests, and metabolizes
  - 10 g/dL to 15 g/dL indicates compromised protein status due to decreased protein or calorie intake
  - ↓10 g/dL indicates possible kwashiorkor
  - Chronic renal failure may be a nonnutritional cause of normal prealbumin levels despite malnutrition
  - Function of prealbumin:
    - Transports portion of thyroxine
    - Transports vitamin A
  - Causes of abnormally low levels of prealbumin:
    - Surgical trauma
    - Stress
    - Inflammation
    - Infection
    - Liver dysfunction

— Carbohydrates: consult with a dietician for the correct amount of carbohydrate necessary for the homeostasis and wound healing for each client.

- Function of carbohydrates:
  - Cellular energy
  - Spares protein
- Deficiency of carbohydrates causes the body to catabolize itself starting with visceral and muscle proteins for energy

— Fats (lipids): consult with a dietician for the correct amount of fat necessary for homeostasis and wound healing for each client.

- Function of fats:
  - Cellular energy
  - Supply essential fatty acids
  - Cell membrane construction
  - Prostaglandin production

• Deficiency of fats causes impaired tissue repair

— Calories required for wound healing are 1500 to 3500 a day

— Water intake required for wound healing is 2000 cc to 2500 cc/day

— Vitamin C (ascorbic acid) 60 mg/day

- Function of vitamin C:
  - Membrane integrity
  - Collagen formation
  - Iron absorption
  - Wound healing
  - Hormone synthesis
- Vitamin C deficiency causes:
  - Impaired healing
  - Capillary fragility
  - Scurvy

— Vitamin A: men require 1000 micrograms/day, women require 800 micrograms/day
  - Function of vitamin A:
    - Collagen synthesis
    - Epithelialization, maintains epithelial tissue
    - Bone growth, reproduction
  - Deficiency of vitamin A causes:
    - Impaired healing
    - Degeneration epithelial tissue, inhibited growth
    - Night blindness
  - Vitamin B_6 (pyridoxine): 1.3 mg/day
    - Function of pyridoxine:
    - Forms coenzyme pyridoxal phosphate (PLP) for energy metabolism
    - Central nervous system function; hemoglobin synthesis
  - Deficiency of vitamin B_6 causes:
    - Dermatitis
    - Weakness
    - Anemia
    - Altered nerve function
  - Vitamin B_{12} (cobalamin): 2.4 micrograms/day
  - Function of Vitamin B_{12}:
    - Antibody and white blood cell formation
    - Cofactors in cellular development
    - Promote enzyme activity
    - Transport/storage of folate
    - Metabolism fatty acids/amino acids
  - Deficiency of Vitamin B_{12} causes impaired immunity
— Folate (folic acid, folacin, PGA): 400 micrograms/day
  - Function of folate is coenzyme metabolism (amino acid synthesis)

- Deficiency of folate causes:
  - Megaloblastic anemia
  - NOTE: many drugs affect folate use by body tissues
- Zinc (Zn): daily requirement for men is 15 mg and for women is 12 mg
- Function of zinc:
  - Cell proliferation & healing
  - Cofactor for enzymes
- Deficiency of zinc causes:
  - Prolonged healing time
  - Anorexia
  - Taste alteration
  - ↓ immunity

— Iron (Fe): daily requirement for men is 10 mg/day and for women is 15 mg/day
— Function of iron:
  - Collagen synthesis
  - Enhances leukocytic bacterial activity
  - Oxygen transport to cells
— Deficiency of iron causes:
  - Leads to risk of local tissue ischemia due to anemia
  - Impaired tensile strength
  - Impaired collagen cross-linkage
— Copper (Cu): 1.5–3.0 mg/day
— Function of copper:
  - Collagen cross-linkage
  - Component of wound healing
  - Nerve fiber protection
— Deficiency of copper causes:
  - Decreased collagen synthesis
  - Bone demineralization and anemia

MULTIDISCIPLINARY PLAN OF CARE RELATIVE TO NUTRITION

- Nutrition plays a critical role in wound healing. All relative members of the multidisciplinary team should be included in the patient's nutrition plan of care.

- Baseline laboratory values should be obtained and retested on admission and every month and in the presence of significant changes with the patient. The following basic laboratory values should be obtained:

  — CBC
  — Prealbumin
  — Serum albumin
  — Electrolyte
  — Creatinine
  — BUN
  — Liver enzymes
  — HgA1c
  — FBS

- Multiple vitamin supplementation is suggested. Centrum Silver or an equivalent in the age 65 and older population and nephrovite in renal failure patients is recommended.

- An additional 500 mg to 1000 mg of vitamin C taken daily by mouth while the wound is open if the patient does not have diabetes mellitus, renal disease, or liver disease is recommended.

- Zinc gluconate or sulfate 110 mg to 220 mg by mouth three times a day may be added if patient has a zinc deficiency or if the patient does not consume animal protein, whole grains, legumes, or eggs in sufficient quantities.

  — Verify with the physician and pharmacist the amount of elemental zinc in each type, and how much the patient actually needs.
  — NOTE: zinc carbonate is a liquid form. Laboratory tests may be performed to confirm zinc deficiency.

— Ferrous gluconate or sulfate dosing is dependent on laboratory findings. The form—tablet, liquid, capsule, soft capsule, timed-release drops, or suspension—is dependent on the patient's ability to ingest the medication.

— NOTE: concurrent administration of more or equal milligrams of vitamin C per 30 mg of elemental iron increases the absorption of oral iron.

— Iron has multiple food interactions that interferes with absorption such as milk, cereals, dietary fiber, tea, coffee, and eggs.

— Iron supplementation may result in a false positive on a stool guaic test.

- Diet orders are required so the patient maintains calories and hydration to support homeostasis and wound healing.

- Height and weight are taken baseline on admission and monthly for the time the wound remains open.

- Food and fluid log is maintained for 72 hours in home health and longer in other levels of care; reevaluate at anytime the wound demonstrates significant decrease in healing or symptoms of infection are present.

- The patient and caregivers should be educated on dietary foods and fluids that enhance healing.

- Documentation in the patient record includes:

  — All education provided

  — Patient and caregiver response to education

  — Provider expectation of patient and caregiver relative to education

  — "Homework" given to the patient

  — Diet log

- Follow-up visits include:

  — Questions about the patient's "homework" progress

  — Questions about how well the patient and caregiver are following the education provided

- Refer the patient to the dietician when:
  - — Prealbumin/albumin levels are less than normal
  - — Nutritional deficiencies are adversely effecting wound outcome
    - Enteral/parenteral feedings are needed
    - Special diets—renal, vegan, diabetic—are needed
- The provider has questions about the patient's nutritional status.
- The wound has not demonstrated healing or progress within the expected time frame even if the laboratory studies are normal and the patient seems to be eating normally.

REFERENCES

1. Acne.com.PharmacologicalTriggers. Available at: www.acne.com/prevention/medications.php. Accessed January 25, 2008.
2. Dermatology. What is Acne? Available at www.skincarephysicians.com/acnenet/acne.html. Accessed January 25, 2008.
3. Bates-Jensen BM, Wethe J. Acute Surgical Wound Management. In: Sussman, C, Bates-Jensen B. *Wound Care A Collaborative Practice Manual for Physical Therapists and Nurses.* Gaithersburg, MD: Aspen Publications; 1998.
4. Lazarus GS, et al. Definitions and guidelines for assessment for wounds and evaluation of healing. *Archives of Dermatology.* April 1994;130(4):489-93.
5. Holloway NM. *Medical-Surgical Care Planning.* 4th ed. Philadelphia, PA: Lippincott Williams & Wilkins; 2003.
6. Baranoski S, Ayello E. *Wound Care Essentials Practice Principles.* Philadelphia, PA: Lippincott Williams & Wilkins; 2004.
7. Payne RL, Martin ML. Defining and classifying skin tears: Need for a common language. *Ostomy Wound Manage.* 1993;39(5):16-20, 22-24, 26.

SUGGESTED READING

Beck FK, Rosenthal TC. Prealbumin: A marker for nutritional evaluation. *American Family Physician.* 65(8):1575–1578.

Bryant RA. *Acute and Chronic Wounds.* St. Louis, MO: Mosby Year Book; 1992.

Diegelmann R, Parks W, Harding K. Research: Pathophysiology of Wound Epithelization. Paper presented at: 2003 Symposium on Advanced Wound Care; April 28, 2003; Las Vegas, NV.

Grodner M, et al. *Foundations and Clinical Applications of Nutrition A Nursing Approach.* 2nd ed. St Louis, MO: Mosby Inc; 2000.

Habif TP, et al. *Skin Disease Diagnosis and Treatment.* St. Louis, MO: Mosby Inc; 2001.

Seidel H, Ball J, Dains J, Benedict GW.. *Mosby's Guide to Physical Examination.* 4th ed. St. Louis, MO: Mosby Inc; 1999.

Stalano-Coico, et al. Wound fluids: A reflection of the state of healing. *Ostomy/Wound Management.* January 2000;46(suppl 1A):85S–93S.

Sussman C, Bates-Jensen B. *Wound Care A Collaborative Practice Manual for Physical Therapists and Nurses.* Gaithersburg, MD: Aspen Publications; 1998.

Support Systems International, Inc. *The Skin, Module 1.* Charleston, SC: Hillenbrand; 1993.

Swartz M. *Textbook of Physical Diagnosis History and Examination.* 3rd ed. Philadelphia, PA: WB Saunders; 1998.

Tierney L, McPhee, S, Papadakis, M. *Current Medical Diagnosis and Treatment.* 37th ed. Stamford, CT: Appleton & Lange; 1998.

White MW, et al. Skin tears in frail elders: A practical approach to prevention. *Geriatric Nursing.* 1994;15(2):95–99.

Voegeli D. The role of emollients in the care of patients with dry skin. *Nursing Standard.* October 2007;22:62–68.

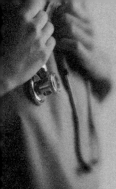

Chapter 3

PRESSURE ULCER ASSESSMENT AND MANAGEMENT PRINCIPLES

KEY POINTS

- Deep tissue necrosis and loss of tissue volume in the pressure ulcer is much greater than what appears as overlying skin damage. This may result in
  — Underestimation of the total length of healing time and the appropriate treatment required for healing.
  — Underestimation of the total problem contributing to the pressure ulcer.
- Muscle and subcutaneous tissues are highly susceptible to pressure injury from either direct or shearing forces on segmental and perforator arteries while cutaneous vessels often benefit from nearby anastomizing vessels.
- Individuals with vascular or neurological abnormalities such as diabetes mellitus or spinal cord injury have increased susceptibility to pressure injury.
- The health-care provider should assess patients for the risk of developing pressure ulcers using a validated tool such as the Braden or Norten scale. Additionally, individualized treatment should be based on the specific patient's needs and risk factors.

PRESSURE ULCERS

Generally pressure ulcers are local areas of tissue trauma over soft tissue where pressure has compressed one area of tissue between a bony prominence and any external surface for a prolonged time period. These ulcers form open sores, are the result of mechanical injury to the skin and underlying tissues, and may or may not have a secretion of pus or other fluid.

- Definition: a pressure ulcer is localized injury to the skin and/or underlying tissue usually over a bony prominence, as a result of pressure, or pressure in combination with shear and/or friction (Figure 3–1). A number of contributing or confounding factors are also associated with pressure ulcers; the significance of these factors is yet to be elucidated.

2007 Staging System for Pressure Ulcers

- The National Pressure Ulcer Advisory Panel (NPUAP) developed a staging system for determining the amount and type of tissue involved in the pressure ulcer as follows:
- The National Pressure Ulcer Advisory Panel (February 2007) has redefined the definition of a pressure ulcer and the stages of pressure ulcers, including the original four stages and adding two stages on deep tissue injury and unstageable pressure ulcers. This work is the culmination of over 5 years of work beginning with the identification of deep tissue injury in 2001.
- The NPUAP staging system (Table 3–1) was defined by Shea in 1975 and provides a name to the amount of anatomical tissue loss. The original definitions were confusing to many clinicians and lead to inaccurate staging of ulcers associated or due to perineal dermatitis and those due to deep tissue injury.

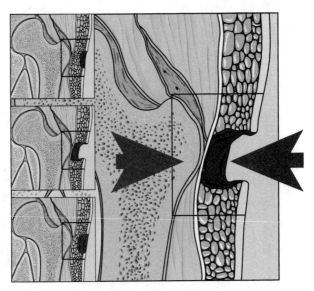

Figure 3–1 NPUAP staging system. (*Continued*)

Formation of a Pressure Sore (Bedsore or Decubitus Ulcer)

Stages of Pressure Sores

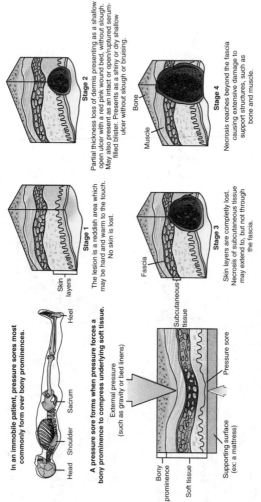

In an immobile patient, pressure sores most commonly form over bony prominences.

Head   Shoulder   Sacrum   Heel

A pressure sore forms when pressure forces a bony prominence to compress underlying soft tissue.

External pressure (such as gravity or bed linens)

Bony prominence

Soft tissue

Pressure sore

Supporting surface (ex: a mattress)

Skin layers

Stage 1
The lesion is a reddish area which may be hard and warm to the touch. No skin is lost.

Stage 2
Partial thickness loss of dermis presenting as a shallow open ulcer with a red pink wound bed, without slough. May also present as an intact or open/ruptured serum-filled blister. Presents as a shiny or dry shallow ulcer without slough or bruising.

Subcutaneous tissue

Fascia

Stage 3
Skin layers are completely lost. Necrosis of subcutaneous tissue may extend to, but not through, the fascia.

Bone

Muscle

Stage 4
Necrosis reaches beyond the fascia causing extensive damage to support structures, such as bone and muscle.

Figure 3–1 NPUAP staging system. (Redrawn from illustration Copyright © 2008 Nucleus Medical Art. All rights reserved. www.nucleusinc.com.)

Table 3-1 NPUAP Pressure Ulcer Stages

Stage I	Intact skin with nonblanchable redness of a localized area usually over a bony prominence. Darkly pigmented skin may not have visible blanching; its color may differ from the surrounding area. The area may be painful, firm, soft, warmer or cooler as compared to adjacent tissue. Stage I may be difficult to detect in individuals with dark skin tones. May indicate "at risk" persons (a heralding sign of risk) (see Figure 3–2).
Stage II	Partial thickness loss of dermis presenting as a shallow open ulcer with a red pink wound bed, without slough. May also present as an intact or open/ruptured serum-filled blister. Presents as a shiny or dry shallow ulcer without slough or bruising. NOTE: this stage should not be used to describe skin tears, tape burns, perineal dermatitis, maceration or excoriation. Bruising indicates suspected deep tissue injury (see Figure 3–3).
Stage III	Full thickness tissue loss. Subcutaneous fat may be visible but bone, tendon, or muscle are not exposed. Slough may be present but does not obscure the depth of tissue loss. May include undermining and tunneling. The depth of a stage III pressure ulcer varies by anatomical location. The bridge of the nose, ear, occiput, and malleolus do not have subcutaneous tissue and stage III ulcers can be shallow. In contrast, areas of significant adiposity can develop extremely deep stage III pressure ulcers. Bone/tendon is not visible or directly palpable (see Figure 3–4).
Stage IV	Full thickness tissue loss with exposed bone, tendon or muscle. Slough or eschar may be present on some parts of the wound bed. Often include undermining and tunneling. The depth of a stage IV pressure ulcer varies by anatomical location. The bridge of the nose, ear, occiput, and malleolus do not have subcutaneous tissue and these ulcers can be shallow. Stage IV ulcers can extend into muscle and/or supporting structures (e.g., fascia, tendon, or joint capsule) making osteomyelitis possible. Exposed bone/tendon is visible or directly palpable (see Figure 3–5).
Unstageable	Full thickness tissue loss in which the base of the ulcer is covered by slough (yellow, tan, gray, green, or brown) and/or eschar (tan, brown or black) in the wound. Until enough slough and/or eschar is removed to expose the base of the wound, the true depth, and therefore stage, cannot be determined. Stable (dry, adherent, intact without erythema or fluctuance) eschar on the heels serves as "the body's natural (biological) cover" and should not be removed.

Source: National Pressure Ulcer Advisory Panel Support Surface Standards Initiative. http://www.npuap.org/pr2.htm

- The proposed definitions were refined by the NPUAP with input from an online evaluation of their face validity, accuracy clarity, succinctness, utility, and discrimination. This process was completed online and provided input to the Panel for continued work. The proposed final definitions were reviewed by a consensus conference and their comments were used to create the final definitions. "NPUAP is pleased to have completed this important task and look forward to the inclusion of these definitions into practice, education, and research,"according to Joyce Black, NPUAP President and Chairperson of the Staging Task Force.

  — For more information, go to http://www.npuap.org or telephone 202-521-6789.

- Suspected Deep Tissue Injury: purple or maroon localized area of discolored intact skin or blood-filled blister due to damage of underlying soft tissue from pressure and/or shear. The area may be preceded by tissue that is painful, firm, mushy, boggy, warmer or cooler as compared to adjacent tissue.

  — Deep tissue injury may be difficult to detect in individuals with dark skin tones. Evolution may include a thin blister over a dark wound bed. The wound may further evolve and become covered by thin eschar. Evolution may be rapid exposing additional layers of tissue even with optimal treatment.[5,6]

- Eschar: black, tan, or brown devitalized or necrotic tissue in the wound bed

- Slough: yellow, tan, gray, green, or brown mucinous tissue that is also devitalized or necrotic

Pressure Ulcer Characteristics

- Location: most often over bony prominences, but may be over soft tissue
- Size: may be any size or depth
- Edema: often present in early stages

- Pain: stage I and II most common
- Stage I, II, III, or IV OR unstageable if wound base cannot be visualized
- With or without necrotic, devitalized tissue
- With or without exudates
- Periwound skin: often involved with edema, induration, temperature, pain, itching, and coloration changes
- Wound edges: varies; may have undermining, tunneling, hypergranulation
- Figures 3–2, 3–3, 3–4, and 3–5 illustrate the characteristics of each pressure ulcer stage.

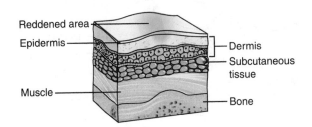

Figure 3–2 Stage 1 pressure ulcer. (From Hess CT. *Wound Care*. 2nd ed. Springhouse, PA: Springhouse Corp; 1998, p. 17.)

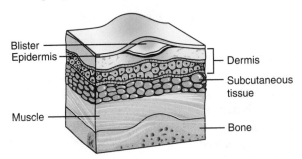

Figure 3–3 Stage 2 pressure ulcer. (From Hess CT. *Wound Care*. 2nd ed. Springhouse, PA: Springhouse Corp; 1998, p. 17.)

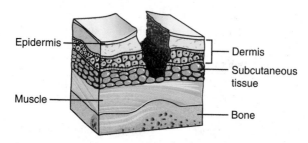

Figure 3–4 Stage 3 pressure ulcer. (From Hess CT. *Wound Care*. 2nd ed. Springhouse, PA: Springhouse Corp; 1998, p. 17.)

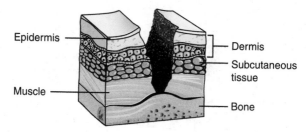

Figure 3–5 Stage 4 pressure ulcer. (From Hess CT. *Wound Care*. 2nd ed. Springhouse, PA: Springhouse Corp; 1998, p. 17.)

Common Locations of Pressure Ulcers

- Scapula
- Iliac crest
- Trochanter
- Sacrum/coccyx
- Ischial tuberosities
- Lateral malleolus
- Lateral edge of foot
- Heel (dorsal or lateral aspect usually more common than plantar surface)
- Bridge of nose

- Occiput
- Ear
- Figure 3–6 shows common locations of pressure ulcers

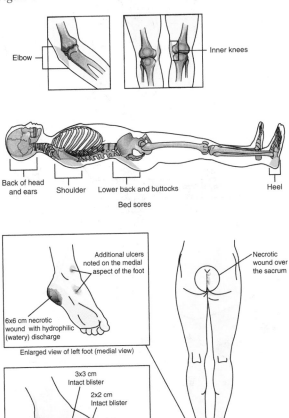

Figure 3–6 Pressure ulcer location. (*Continued*)

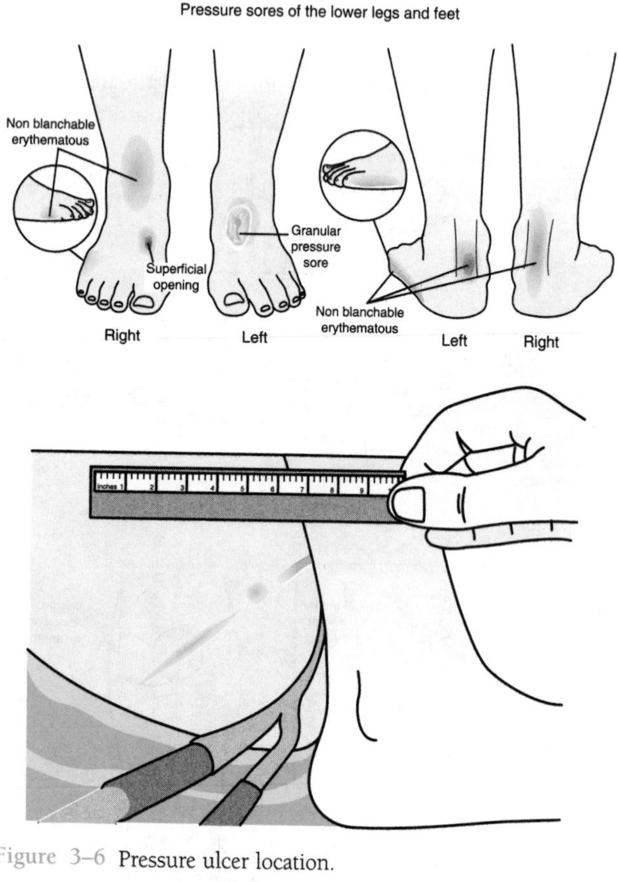

Pressure sores of the lower legs and feet

Non blanchable erythematous

Superficial opening

Granular pressure sore

Non blanchable erythematous

Right   Left   Left   Right

Figure 3–6 Pressure ulcer location.

Risk Factors for Pressure Ulcer Development

* Bed rest—either medically required or patient preferred—especially if chronically ill, obese, or very thin
* Dehydration
* Diabetes mellitus (due to potential for loss of sensation)

- Diminished awareness of pain
- Fractures
- Corticosteroid therapy
- Inadequate nutritional status (especially malnutrition)
- Immunosuppression
- Incontinence (urinary and/or fecal or both as the skin in contact with incontinence becomes more fragile)
- Cognitive impairments:
  — Altered consciousness levels
  — Coma
  — Sedation
  — Confusion
  — Alzheimer disease or other dementias
  — Depression (chronic or acute)
- Multiple trauma sites/systems
- Paralysis (partial or complete)
- Inadequate circulation (venous and/or arterial, or both)
- Significant obesity or significant thinness
- History of previous pressure ulcers

Contributing Factors for Pressure Ulcer Development

Nursing Tip
The goal of the nurse is to evaluate, mitigate, or manage the factors that contribute to pressure ulcer development in order to prevent the breakdown of the skin.

- Pressure: immobility, inactivity, and loss of sensory perception affect the duration and intensity of pressure.
  — 12–32 mmHg capillary closing pressure,
  — Low intensity of pressure over a long period of time, OR

— High intensity of pressure over a short period of time

- According to one study, individuals who have greater than 50 spontaneous movements a night did not develop pressure ulcers while those with 20 or fewer movements developed pressure ulcers.[1]

- Friction: "the rubbing of one body against another; the resistance which any body meets with in moving over another body" (Oxford English Dictionary). Friction is a contributing factor to the development of pressure ulcers that may prolong the healing of any wound.

— Friction reduces the tissue tolerance to pressure by abrading and damaging the epidermal and upper dermal skin layers.

— When friction exists with pressure, ulcers are produced at lower pressure levels.

— Friction in conjunction with shear contributes to the development of sacral and/or coccygeal pressure ulcers in patients positioned in semi-Fowler's position.

— Friction involves the epidermal and dermal layers.

- Shear: "the stress called into play in a body which undergoes a kind of strain consisting in a movement of planes of a body that are parallel to a particular plane" (Oxford English Dictionary). Shear acts with a parallel force that causes tissue ischemia through lateral blood vessel displacement that results in blood flow disruption or impediment.

— Shear twists and stretches tissue and blood vessels at bony tissue interfaces and therefore affects deeper tissue structures and deep blood vessels.

— Semi-Fowler's bed position is the most common cause of shear.

— This effect is also the reason many pressure ulcers over a bony prominence are substantially larger than the bony prominence over which they occur.

— Gravity plus friction equals shear.

— Shear affects the deep fascial level and bony prominences.

- Moisture: "the liquid part or constituent of a body" (*Oxford English Dictionary*). Moisture removes protective skin oils from the skin therefore creating more friable skin.
  — Moisture also interacts with friction.
  — Mild to moderate moisture (diaphoresis, fecal or urinary incontinence, wound exudate) causes an increase of shearing force and friction.
  — Urinary incontinence exposes the skin to excess moisture as well as chemical damage.
  — Fecal incontinence adds to the risk stated above by adding bacteria and bowel enzymes.
  — Evaluate cause of urinary and fecal incontinence (may be dietary, mechanical, environmental, or physical).
  — Implement a bladder training program.
  — Constant moisture causes maceration (water logging of the tissues) that softens connective tissue and erodes the epidermis making it more susceptible to damage.
- Blood Pressure (BP)
  — When systolic BP is below 100 and diastolic BP is below 60, wound healing may take longer or may be diminished. The patient may be at increased risk of developing pressure ulcers over areas at risk.
- Mobility: "the ability to move or to be moved; capacity for movement or change of place" (*Oxford English Dictionary*).
  — Less exercise or decreased mobility may cause longer healing times or may result in diminished healing increasing the patient's risk of developing pressure ulcers over areas of risk.
- Mechanical damage or epidermal stripping: the epidermal layer is actually stripped away.
  — The primary cause is caregivers (health-care and others) when they remove dressings or medical adhesives and do NOT use the push-pull technique—the tissue is pushed away from the adhesive as the adhesive is gently being pulled away from the tissue simultaneously.

- Elevated temperature: especially in the elderly; wound healing may take longer or diminished wound healing may result when there is alteration in the body temperature for long periods of time.
- Medications: may prolong or diminish wound healing.
  — Evaluate all medications (efficacy)
  — Corticosteroids (withhold for 4–5 days after ulcer appearance if possible)
  — Antibacterials
  — Antihypertensives
  — Analgesics
  — Antidepressants
  — Antihistamines
  — Oncological chemotherapeutics
- Tobacco use: higher incidence of pressure ulcer development and increased time for healing with number of packs per day smoked.
- Psychological status: must be evaluated as it may diminish or slow wound healing. Evaluate the patient's
  — Motivation
  — Emotional energy
  — Emotional stress
- Additional factors that increase the risk for nonhealing or prolonged healing of pressure ulcers:
  — Heredity
  — Malignancies
  — Substance abuse
  — Radiation therapy
  — Oncological chemotherapy
  — Foreign bodies in or around the wound such as joint replacement hardware and sutures
  — Inadequately managed wound exudate

— Inability to control, reduce, or eliminate other risk factors
— Iatrogenic factors

NURSING PROTOCOLS FOR PRESSURE ULCER PREVENTION AND TREATMENT

* Pressure reduction
* Pressure relief
* Turning schedule according to patient needs, NOT protocol (only full body change of position completely relieves pressure)
  — 30-degree lateral, NOT side-lying position
* Pillow bridging is placed:
  — Under the legs to elevate the heels off any surface such as a mattress or wheelchair foot rest
  — Between the ankles
  — Between the knees
  — Behind the back (some controversy continues but recommended at this time)
  — Under the head with the neck supported (with the least amount of pressure at the occiput)
* Exercise and mobility (active and passive range of motion)
* Do not use donuts or inflatable rings
* Do not directly massage the affected area
* Restorative nursing program
  — Include nursing assistants and home health aides in the plan of care (POC)

Friction Prevention and Treatment

* Skin sealants and skin barriers (alcohol- or nonalcohol-based)
* Moisturizers and skin lubricants (high water content)
* Elbow and heel protectors

- Corn starch sprinkled on the bed linens (NEVER use talcum powder that may cause skin abrading)
- Appropriate repositioning techniques
- Restorative nursing program
    — Include nursing assistants and home health aides in the POC

Shear Prevention and Treatment

- 30-degree head elevation for short periods of time (prevent the patient from sliding down in the bed)
- Foot board
- Knee gatch
- Use of lift sheets with repositioning to reduce dragging of any body surfaces with the position change
- Heel protection (NOT foam pads or dressings but actually elevating the heels off mattress; use of special heel devices)
- Specialty mattresses and beds (not reimbursable by Medicare unless a wound is present)
- Appropriate repositioning techniques
- Restorative nursing program
    — Include nursing assistants and home health aides in the POC

Mechanical Damage and Epidermal Stripping Prevention and Treatment

- Porous tape without tension; apply skin barrier wipe before applying tape if fragile skin is present
- Careful adhesive removal; push-pull technique with ALL adhesives
- Skin sealants and skin barrier wipes (alcohol and nonalcohol based)
- Other securing methods such as Montgomery straps, non-allergic tape, hydrocolloid under tape, and stretch net dressings

- Enzymes
  — Evaluate cause of fecal and urinary incontinence (may be dietary, mechanical, environmental, or physical.) Correct whenever possible to avoid caustic effects on the skin. If unable to correct use petrolatum or zinc-oxide–based skin protectants in periwound area.
- Restorative nursing program
  — Include nursing assistants and home health aides in the POC

Moisture Prevention and Treatment

- Absorbent powders (NEVER talcum powder as it is abrasive)
- Skin sealants and skin barrier wipes (alcohol- and nonalcohol-based)
- Dressing changes as necessary to keep moisture off the skin
- Use of absorbent cotton materials in skin folds
- Restorative nursing program
  — Include nursing assistants and home health aides in the POC

Immobility Prevention and Treatment

- Encourage patient independence in all activities as tolerated
- Active range of motion (AROM) with all dependent activities
- Specific exercises such as straight leg raises and ankle pump exercises
- Physical therapy or occupational therapy referral as indicated for muscle reeducation and establishing a rehabilitative program
- Restorative nursing program
  — Include nursing assistants and home health aides in the POC

Increased Blood Pressure Prevention and Treatment

- Treat the cause of high blood pressure
- Teach patient and caregiver how to monitor blood pressure

- Diet and fluid log determines any potential causes of blood pressure disparity
- Medication log determines any potential causes of blood pressure disparity
- Pre- and postactivity blood pressure determines any potential causes of blood pressure disparity
- Consider dietitian referral to educate patient about diet to control high blood pressure
- Consider when blood pressure medications are administered and change administration time as appropriate
- Restorative nursing program
  — Include nursing assistants and home health aides in the POC

Increased Temperature Prevention and Treatment

- Manage symptoms with type and amount of clothing, diet and fluid intake, and medications
- Treat cause of temperature elevation including evaluating hydration status
- Diet and fluid log to determine any potential causes of temperature disparity
- Consider dietitian referral to educate patient about diet to control and prevent increased temperature
- Medication log to determine any potential causes of temperature disparity
- Restorative nursing program
  — Include nursing assistants and home health aides in the POC

Protocols for Tobacco Cessation

- Educate and support efforts to quit tobacco
- Provide smoking cessation literature
- Refer to appropriate smoking cessation program
- Refer to appropriate support groups

Protocols for Improving Psychological Status

- Encourage and support patient and caregiver
- Relaxation techniques for patient
- Activity for patient
- Medical social worker and chaplain referral
- Psychiatric referral
- Restorative nursing program
  — Include nursing assistants and home health aides in the POC

BODY FUNCTIONS THAT IMPAIR WOUND HEALING

Evaluate each client with a wound for body functions that contribute to impaired wound healing. Focus on treatment, stabilization, and prevention.

- Respiratory system: oxygen deficits and carbon dioxide excesses can impair wound healing. Counteract this by implementing
  — Occupational therapy referral for energy conservation
  — Restorative nursing program
    ▪ Include nursing assistants and home health aides in the POC
  — Pulse oximetry (include in POC)
  — Medication management systems
  — Medical social worker referral for psychosocial interventions and long-term planning

- Cardiovascular system: circulation and perfusion to and from wounded areas, impaired waste removal, and bleeding deficiencies can impair wound healing. Treatment includes:
  — Restorative nursing program
    ▪ Include nursing assistants and home health aides in the POC

- — Occupational therapy referral for activities of daily living (ADLs) and energy conservation
- — Home rehabilitation program (CHHAs)
- — Medication management systems
- — MSW referral for psychosocial interventions, long-term planning
- Gastrointestinal system: malabsorption and the acidity or alkalinity of secretions and excretions can impair wound healing. Treatment includes
  - — Nursing assistant and home health aide plan of care includes nutrition and meal preparation and reporting of patient intake at each meal
  - — Restorative nursing program (bowel retraining)
    - Include nursing assistant and home health aide in the POC for patient assistance with training, reporting, and recording of results of bowel training program
  - — Referral to dietician
  - — Speech language pathologist and physical therapist referral for swallowing evaluation
  - — Medical social worker referral for assistance in reducing food costs and providing psychosocial interventions (especially with incontinence issues)
- Musculoskeletal system: immobility and decreased position changes can lead to decreased wound healing. The patient may benefit by
  - — Physical therapy and occupational therapy referral
    - Include physical therapy aide, nursing assistant, and home health aides in the POC for patient assistance with training, reporting, and recording of results
  - — Home rehabilitation program (CHHAs)
  - — Restorative nursing program
  - — Include nursing assistant and home health aide in the POC
  - — Medical social worker referral for durable medical equipment costs, psychosocial interventions, and long-term planning

- Genitourinary system: moisture and chemical irritation, faulty collagen deposition, and impaired waste removal may impair wound healing. Treatment includes:

— Correct barrier product use
  - Petrolatum based moisture barriers
  - Zinc Oxide based barriers
  - Skin barrier wipes (alcohol- and nonalcohol-based)
  - Hydrocolloid on wounds as appropriate

— Bladder retraining program

— AVOID adult plastic diapers whenever possible. Diapers in an adult patient reduce continence. Diapers should only be used if a consistent bladder program has not been successful and has been evaluated for cause of lack of success.

— AVOID continuous Foley catheterization of the bladder EXCEPT in cases of retention. Foley catheterization may be necessary for short term (2–4 weeks) ONLY if the wounded skin cannot be kept free of urinary incontinence in any other manner.

— Restorative nursing program (bladder retraining)
  - Include nursing assistants and home health aides in the POC for patient assistance with training, reporting, and recording of results of bladder training program

— Occupational therapy referral for assistance with ADLs and assistive devices

— Certified wound ostomy continence nurse referral for containment devices and skin treatment

— Medical social worker referral for assistance with costs of products and psychosocial interventions (especially with incontinence)

- Neurologic system: impaired awareness and sensation impairs wound healing.
Treatment includes:

— Evaluation of all skin folds especially on affected limbs for rashes and tears

— Use antifungal topical treatments such as Lotrimin 1% with physician order and supervision

— Use acetic acid 0.25% on fungal rash; cools the itching and burning

— Do not cover rashes with dressings.

  ▪ If clothing is necessary in the area of the rash, advise wearing 100% cotton.

  ▪ Clothing and bedding must be washed in hot water and white household vinegar added to the rinse cycle (1–2 cups for large loads).

  ▪ If using antifungals for foot rashes, the shoes must be cleansed with acetic acid solution, allowed to dry in direct sunlight, and recleansed after every use.

  ▪ Use of an over-the-counter antifungal foot powder in the shoes is also advisable.

— Physical therapy and occupational therapy referral

— Home rehabilitation program

— Restorative nursing program

  ▪ Include nursing assistants and home health aides in the POC for patient assistance with training, reporting, and recording of results

— Medical social worker for assistance with cost of products and durable medical equipment, psychosocial interventions, and long-term planning

— Speech language pathologist referral for communication and swallowing.

• Endocrine system: infection and basement membrane thickening retards healing. Treatment includes

— Evaluation of blood sugars; fasting 90 mg/dL to 110 mg/dL is the target range according to the American Association of Clinical Endocrinologists (ACE) (http://www.aace.com/)

— Medical social worker referral for assistance with costs of products and durable medical equipment, psychosocial interventions, and long-term planning

— Diabetes nurse specialist referral

— Dietitian referral

PRESSURE ULCER TREATMENT

- Common guidelines to treat pressure ulcers include:
- Agency for Healthcare Research and Quality (AHRQ) guidelines for treatment regimens. Refer to Internet resources at end of this chapter for more guidelines and patient and caregiver information
- Wound Ostomy Continence Nurses (WOCN) guidance on OASIS Skin and Wound Status MO Items for Home Health; refer to www.wocn.org.
- Prevention
- Timely reassessments and evaluations of treatments
- Skin cleansing
- Minimize skin drying
- Eliminate or minimize massage of affected areas
- Eliminate or minimize pressure. (Evaluate all support surfaces for "bottoming out" at each visit and correct when present.)
- Eliminate or minimize friction and shear
- Eliminate or minimize exposure to incontinence, exudate, and perspiration
- Assess and treat all risk factors, pain, and psychological states
- Educate caregivers and patients on prevention, signs and symptoms to report, and treatment
- The principles of wound care and treatment:
    - Remove foreign bodies and necrotic tissue
    - Identify and control infection
    - Absorb excess exudates
    - Maintain moist wound bed
    - Fill in dead space of undermining, tunnels, or sinus tracts

— Keep the wound bed warm
— Protect the wound from trauma and microbial invasion

Pressure Ulcer Treatment Relative to Stage

- Stage I
  — Educate nursing assistants and home health aides
  — Inspect all bony prominences during waking hours (every shift, twice daily, or more often)
  — Turning schedule every 2 hours to reduce pressure
  — Heels off mattress while in bed
  — NO massaging of the ulcer or periwound skin
  — Dressing only if in an area of moisture or friction as in incontinence or the heels
  — Apply a nonadherent, protective dressing
  — Use extreme care with any cleansing of ulcer
  — Instruct patient and family in basic skin care and repositioning while in bed and while seated
  — Avoid use of diapers if ulcer is in area of incontinence whenever possible
  — Use appropriate lifting and positioning techniques
  — Avoid use of soap to all dry skin areas
  — Lotion may be used in bath water
  — Apply moisturizers twice daily to entire body
  — Inspect and evaluate shoe gear for evidence of improper fit

- Stage II
  — Educate nursing assistants and home health aides
  — Inspect all bony prominences during waking hours (every shift, twice daily, or more often)
  — Turning schedule every 2 hours to reduce pressure
  — Heels off mattress while in bed
  — Foot cradle if ulcer is on foot, toe, or heel

— NO massaging of the ulcer or periwound skin
— Instruct patient and family in basic skin care and repositioning while in bed and while seated
— Use appropriate lifting and positioning techniques
— Avoid use of soap to all dry skin areas
— Lotion may be used in bath water instead of soap
— Apply moisturizers twice daily to entire body
— Inspect and evaluate shoe gear for evidence of improper fit
— Evaluate nutritional and hydration status; change plan of care as appropriate
— Ulcer treatment (NOT applicable for heel blisters):
  ▪ Cleanse gently with normal saline (NS)
  ▪ Cover with hydrocolloid
  ▪ Appropriate application of any hydrocolloid requires that a minimum of 1.0 cm of intact skin at the wound edge is under the dressing
  ▪ Change every 3 to 5 days and as needed when leaking, peeling, or contamination with incontinence
— Heel blister treatment:
  ▪ If skin on heel is intact, if heel is elevated off mattress, and leg is elevated when patient is in chair then no dressing is needed
  ▪ If skin is open:
    ○ Cleanse gently with normal saline
    ○ Cover with nonstick, nonwoven gauze
    ○ Instruct patient and family regarding:
      • Proper handwashing
      • Report signs and symptoms of infection
      • Wound care
      • Nutrition and hydration principles
      • Prevention of additional pressure ulcers
      • Proper transfer techniques

- Stage III
  - Educate nursing assistants and home health aides
  - Inspect all bony prominences during waking hours (every shift, twice daily, or more often)
  - Turning schedule every 2 hours to reduce pressure
  - Heels off mattress while in bed
  - Foot cradle if ulcer is on foot, toe, or heel
  - NO massaging of the ulcer or periwound skin
  - Instruct patient and family in basic skin care and repositioning while in bed and while seated
  - Use appropriate lifting and positioning techniques
  - Avoid use of soap to all dry skin areas
  - Lotion may be used in bath water instead of soap
  - Apply moisturizers twice daily to entire body
  - Inspect and evaluate shoe gear for evidence of improper fit
  - Evaluate nutritional and hydration status; change POC as appropriate
  - Limit time up in chair if ulcer is on sitting surface (usually 1 hour; 1–3 times per day)
  - Ulcer treatment:
    - Gently cleanse with normal saline (wound cleanser with surfactant if exudate is tenacious)
    - Apply hydrogel directly to wound or to primary dressing and avoid product contact with intact periwound skin
    - Cover with dry dressing
    - Change every day to twice daily depending on amount of exudate
    - If large amounts of exudate (more than 50% of secondary dressing is saturated in less than 24 hours) do not use hydrogel but apply calcium alginate; keep alginate in contact with wounded skin only to prevent desiccation

- Cover with dry dressing
- Change daily, every other day, or less often depending on amount of exudate
- Instruct patient and family regarding:
  - Proper handwashing
  - Signs and symptoms of infection to report
  - Wound care
  - Nutrition and hydration principles
  - Prevention of additional pressure ulcers
  - Proper transfer techniques

- Stage IV
  — Educate nursing assistants and home health aides
  — Inspect all bony prominences during waking hours (every shift, twice daily, or more often)
  — Turning schedule every 2 hours to reduce pressure
  — Heels off mattress while in bed
  — Foot cradle if ulcer is on foot, toe, heel
  — NO massaging of the ulcer or periwound skin
  — Instruct patient and family in basic skin care and repositioning while in bed and while seated
  — Use appropriate lifting and positioning techniques
  — Avoid use of soap to all dry skin areas
  — Lotion may be used in bath water instead of soap
  — Apply moisturizers twice daily to entire body
  — Inspect and evaluate shoe gear for evidence of improper fit
  — Evaluate nutritional and hydration status; change plan of care as appropriate
  — Limit time up in chair if ulcer is on sitting surface (usually 1 hour; 1–3 times per day)
  — Ulcer treatment:
    - Clean gently with normal saline (wound cleanser with surfactant, if exudate is tenacious)

- Apply hydrogel directly to wound or to primary dressing and avoid product contact with intact periwound skin
- Cover with dry dressing
- Change daily to twice daily depending on amount of exudate
- If large amounts of exudate (more than 50% of secondary dressing is saturated in less than 24 hours) do not use hydrogel but apply calcium alginate
- Keep alginate in contact with wounded skin only to prevent desiccation
- Cover with dry dressing
- Change every day or every other day
- Instruct patient and family regarding:
  - Proper handwashing
  - Signs and symptoms of infection to report
  - Wound care
  - Nutrition and hydration principles
  - Prevention of additional pressure ulcers
  - Proper transfer techniques

SUPPORT SURFACES

Support surfaces are used to control pressure and thus are a major component of treatment and prevention of pressure ulcers. Some surfaces reduce friction, shear, control moisture, and inhibit bacterial proliferation. These devices are available in a multitude of shapes and sizes for use on beds, in chairs, and on the patient's limbs (Box 3–1).

According to the National Pressure Ulcer Advisory Panel Support Surfaces Standards Initiative the following standards are recommended for use relative to support surfaces:[2]

- The terms "static" and "dynamic" refer to clearly different conditions or states of activity. In the world of support surfaces, however, the initial descriptive intent of these words changed and came to mean "nonpowered," and "powered," respectively.

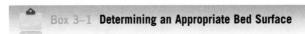

Box 3–1 Determining an Appropriate Bed Surface

Prevention or treatment of stage I or II with one sleep surface impaired:

- Alternating pressure pad with 6 inches or greater of medical grade foam

- No donuts or rings

Treatment of stage III or IV with one sleep surface impaired:

- May use static mattress, overlay, or dynamic mattress

- Limit sitting time if wound is on the ischial tuberosity

- No donuts or rings

Treatment of flap, graft, burn, or stage II with two or three sleep surfaces impaired:

- May use dynamic, low air loss, or air fluidized mattress or bed

- Reduce amount of sitting time if wound is on the ischial tuberosity

- No donuts or rings

Treatment of stage III or IV with two or three sleep surfaces impaired:

- May use low air loss or air-fluidized bed

- Limit amount of sitting time

- No donuts or rings

Any patient who has a wound on a sitting surface—or is at risk of developing one—and who will be sitting for periods of time requires an appropriate pressure redistribution device on all sitting surfaces.

All support surfaces should be assessed for "bottoming out" during each shift and each visit. Patients and caregivers should be educated about how to check this.

- The word "pressure" describes a force over an area. Pressure redistribution supersedes "pressure reduction" and "pressure relief."
- A support surface is a specialized device for pressure redistribution designed for management of tissue loads, microclimate, and/or other therapeutic functions (Tables 3–2, 3–3).
- Dynamic versus static
  - Dynamic surfaces alternate inflation and deflation. Some devices accomplish this with only the force of the individual's breathing, others may require stronger patient movements, and some are programmed to change with the passage of time.
  - Static surfaces maintain a constant inflation (by gel, foam, or water) that molds to the body surface spreading the pressure load over a large area, whereas pressure ulcers encompass a small area.
- Features of support surfaces (Tables 3–4, 3–5)
  - A feature is a functional component of a support surface that can be used alone or in combination with other features.
- Types of devices
  - Foam overlays: commonly used for pressure redistribution. Characteristics include:
    - Base height and thickness (height from base to top). This varies with various products (even from the same manufacturer).
    - Two inches of medical grade foam are for comfort only and do not reduce or relieve pressure.
    - Three to four inches may reduce pressure if the patient is not overweight and the surface is medical grade.
    - Important to validate what loads (weight amount) the manufacturer is allowed to state the device is capable of holding.
    - Density of the foam material (ability to support patient's weight).

Table 3–2 Physical Concepts Related to Support Surfaces

Term	Definition
Friction (Frictional Force)	The resistance to motion in a parallel direction relative to the common boundary of two surfaces.
Coefficient of Friction	A measurement of the amount of friction existing between two surfaces.
Envelopment	The ability of a support surface to conform, fit, or mold around irregularities in the body.
Fatigue	The reduced capacity of a surface or its components to perform as specified. This change may be the result of intended or unintended use and/or prolonged exposure to chemical, thermal, or physical forces.
Force	A push-pull vector with magnitude (quantity) and direction (pressure, shear) that is capable of maintaining or altering the position of a body.
Immersion	Depth of penetration (sinking) into a support surface.
Life Expectancy	The defined period of time during which a product is able to effectively fulfill its designated purpose.
Mechanical Load	Force distribution acting on a surface.
Pressure	The force per unit area exerted perpendicular to the plane of interest.
Pressure Redistribution	The ability of a support surface to distribute load over the contact areas of the human body. The term replaces prior terminology of pressure reduction and pressure relief surfaces.
Pressure Reduction	This term is no longer used to describe classes of support surfaces. The term used is pressure redistribution (see above).
Pressure Relief	This term is no longer used to describe classes of support surfaces. The term used is pressure redistribution (see above).
Shear (Shear Stress)	The force per unit area exerted parallel to the plane of interest.
Shear Strain	Distortion or deformation of tissue as a result of shear stress.

Source: Reference 2, pages 1–2.

Table 3–3 **Components of Support Surfaces**

Term	Definition
Air	A low density fluid with minimal resistance to flow.
Cell/Bladder	A means of encapsulating a support medium.
Viscoelastic Foam	A type of porous polymer material that conforms in proportion to the applied weight. The air exits and enters the foam cells slowly which allows the material to respond slower than a standard elastic foam (memory foam).
Elastic Foam	A type of porous polymer material that conforms in proportion to the applied weight. Air exits and enters the foam cells more rapidly, due to greater density (nonmemory).
Closed Cell Foam	A nonpermeable structure in which there is a barrier between cells, preventing gases or liquids from passing through the foam.
Open Cell Foam	A permeable structure in which there is no barrier between cells, and gases or liquids can pass through the foam.
Gel	A semisolid system consisting of a network of solid aggregates, colloidal dispersions or polymers which may exhibit elastic properties. (Can range from a hard gel to a soft gel).
Pad	A cushion-like mass of soft material used for comfort, protection, or positioning.
Viscous Fluid	A fluid with a relatively high resistance to flow of the fluid.
Elastomer	Any material that can be repeatedly stretched to at least twice its original length, and upon release the stretch will return to approximately its original length.
Solid	A substance that does not flow perceptibly under stress. Under ordinary conditions retains its size and shape.
Water	A moderate density fluid with moderate resistance to flow.

Source: Reference 2, page 3.

Table 3-4   Features of Support Surfaces

Terms	Definition
Air Fluidized	A feature of a support surface that provides pressure redistribution via a fluid-like medium created by forcing air through beads as characterized by immersion and envelopment.
Alternating Pressure	A feature of a support surface that provides pressure redistribution via cyclic changes in loading *and unloading* as characterized by frequency, duration, amplitude, and rate of change parameters.
Lateral Rotation	A feature of a support surface that provides rotation about a longitudinal axis as characterized by degree of patient turn, duration, and frequency.
Low Air Loss	A feature of a support surface that provides a flow of air to assist in managing the heat and humidity (microclimate) of the skin.
Zone	A segment with a single pressure redistribution capability.
Multizoned Surface	A surface in which different segments can have different pressure redistribution capabilities.

Source: Reference 2, page 4.

- Indentation load deflection (ILD) (compressibility, conformability of foam, and foam's ability to distribute the mechanical load)
- Contours (the surface description such as convoluted, slashed, flat, or textured)
— Static air-filled overlays: interconnected cells in the device offer support when inflated
  - Available for chair or bed use; for short- or long-term use
  - Vast majority redistribute pressure
  - Proper inflation is an absolute necessity

Table 3–5 Categories of Support Surfaces

Term	Definition
Reactive Support Surface	A powered or nonpowered support surface with the capability to change its load distribution properties only in response to applied load.
Active Support Surface	A powered support surface with the capability to change its load distribution properties, with or without applied load.
Integrated Bed System	A bed frame and support surface that are combined into a single unit whereby the surface is unable to function separately.
Nonpowered	Any support surface not requiring or using external sources of energy for operation, (Energy = DC or AC).
Powered	Any support surface requiring or using external sources of energy for operation, (Energy = DC or AC).
Overlay	An additional support surface designed to be placed directly on top of an existing surface.
Mattress	A support surface designed to be placed directly on the existing bed frame.

Source: Reference 2, page 5.

— Alternating air-filled mattress overlays: inflation and deflation occurs on an alternating basis with the intent of preventing constant pressure against the skin.
  ▪ MAY enhance blood flow
  ▪ Proper inflation is an absolute necessity
— Gel or water-filled mattress overlays: offer pressure redistribution and are easy to clean while requiring little maintenance. Gel is also used as a mattress replacement in some settings. Gel-filled cushions are also available for chairs.

— Mattress replacements: include foam, gel, combination fillings, and air.

Most are covered with bacteriostatic material but few studies exist that attest to the long-term efficacy and ability of these coverings to control infection.

— Low air-loss mattress replacements: many of these are supported directly on the bed frame, replacing the existing mattress. Most are easy to set up and take down and are therefore used in a variety of health-care settings.

— Low air-loss specialty beds: provide a more even distribution of the patient's weight over a sequence of air-filled pillows. The source of the air is a pumping motor that allows dry air to flow between the patient and the surface. This dry air controls moisture and heat buildup. It is important to know the patient's height, weight, and (often) the body-fat distribution to obtain the appropriate bed.

— Air-fluidized specialty beds: a pump distributes air through silicone-coated microspheres that are separated from the patient by a monofilament sheet. The general feeling is one of floating. These beds are often very heavy and may cause the wound to dry out.

Reimbursement for Support Surfaces in Home Health

- Covered under Medicare Part B (DME) if patient has Part B coverage
- Must be multiple stage IIs, stage III, or stage IV pressure ulcer
- Must be located on trunk of body
- Patient must be living in his or her permanent residence

Positioning Guidelines

- Proper patient positioning can reduce the risk and further development of pressure ulcers (Figures 3–7 and 3–8).

- Risk for pressure ulcer development is greater with sitting than lying down
  - Gravitational force creates greater body weight over smaller surface with seated activities than when flat in bed (more surface to disperse pressures when flat in bed)
- Emphasis on proper positioning includes:
  - Posture
  - Alignment
  - Avoidance of sitting on pressure ulcers or reddened areas
  - Anterior thighs
    - Horizontal
    - Distributes weight evenly along posterior surfaces
    - If knees are higher than hips, body weight shifts to the ischial tuberosities that increase pressure risk

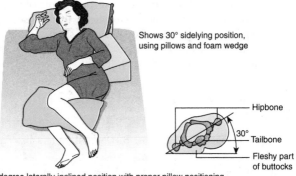

Shows 30° sidelying position, using pillows and foam wedge

Hipbone

30° Tailbone

Fleshy part of buttocks

30-degree laterally inclined position with proper pillow positioning

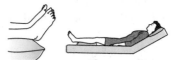

Proper heel placement   Head of bed elevation limited to 30° or less

Figure 3–7 Positioning. (From Maklebust JA, Sieggreen M. *Pressure Ulcers Guidelines for Prevention and Nursing Management.* 3rd ed. Springhouse, PA: Springhouse Corp; 2001.)

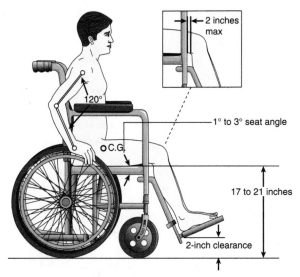

Figure 3–8 Wheelchair positioning. (From Maklebust JA, Sieggreen M. *Pressure Ulcers Guidelines for Prevention and Nursing Management*. 3rd ed. Springhouse, PA: Springhouse Corp; 2001.)

— Reduce risk of pressure on ischial tuberosities by keeping neutral position of:
  ▪ Ankles
  ▪ Elbows
  ▪ Forearms
  ▪ Wrists
— Knees should not rub together; keep them separated
  ▪ Keep seat angle with knees no higher than buttocks to keep ischial and sacral pressure at a minimum to reduce incidence of pressure ulcers
• Repositioning
— Every 15 minutes for individuals able to reposition independently

— If patient has the upper body strength, educate to do push-ups every 15 minutes to reestablish buttocks and sacral blood flow
— If patient does not have upper body strength:
  ▪ Lean forward toward the thighs to reduce pressure over the ischial tuberosities (from 189 mmHg to 34 mmHg and on the ischium from 114 mmHg to 33 mmHg).[3]
  ▪ Chair sitting for those unable to reposition themselves should be limited to 1 hour at a time, then the patient placed back in bed.[4]

• All patients who are at risk should have pressure redistribution devices in the chairs in which they are sitting at all times.

• All pressure redistribution devices for sitting surfaces should be evaluated for "bottoming out" minimally at least each shift and twice daily (Figure 3–9).
  — Patients and caregivers require education in how to perform this and return demonstrations should be documented in every level of care before discharge to the next level of care.
  — Patient and a caregiver must minimally be knowledgeable concerning the following regarding support devices:
    ▪ Device function
    ▪ Cost or share of cost of the device
    ▪ Manufacturer of the device
    ▪ Responsible party for maintaining the device
    ▪ Contact information if there are any problems with the function of the device
    ▪ Responsible party for the maintenance of any device amenities such as pads, covers, buzzers, and whistles
    ▪ Location of instruction manual
    ▪ Warranty information
    ▪ Cleaning schedule

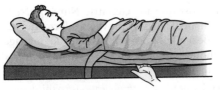

Slide hand (palm up and fingers flat) under support surface, just under pressure point. Do not flex fingers.

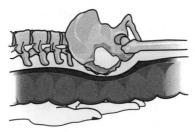

With good support, the patient's bony prominence cannot be felt with flat hand when the patient is in a "worst-case" position (i.e. head of bed is elevated 30°, patient is side-lying on greater trochanter, etc.). Copyright, 1989. Used with permission of Gaymar Industries, Inc.

Figure 3–9 Checking for pressure points.

INTERNET RESOURCES

- **European Pressure Ulcer Advisory Panel** provides information on how countries in Europe manage pressure ulcers as well as European research on the subject.

    —http://www.epuap.org/

- **University of Southern California/Rancho Pressure Ulcer Prevention Project** provides information on rehabilitation, spinal cord injury, and paraplegia/quadriplegia including graphics of pressure ulcers.

    —http://www.usc.edu/programs/pups/articles-in-depth/stages-of-pressure-ulcers.html

- The Hartford Institute for Geriatric Nursing, New York University School of Nursing provides information on incidence, prevalence of pressure ulcers and management options including rationale for using the Braden Scale for Predicting Pressure Sore Risk.

  —http://www.hartfordign.org/publications/trythis/issue05.pdf

- National Institute for Clinical Evidence provides a booklet on pressure ulcer assessment, risk, and prevention.

  —http://www.nice.org.uk/nicemedia/pdf/clinicalguideline-pressuresoreguidancenice.pdf

- Wound, Ostomy, Continence Nurse Society provides list of educational organizations with programs leading to certification as WOCN, policy statements, pressure ulcer guidelines and annual national conferences as well as regional seminars.

  —http:///www.wocn.org

- American Academy of Wound Management is a national interdisciplinary organization with national conferences and list of requirements for certification as a CW healthcare professional.

  —http://www.aawm.org/

- Queensland Government Pressure Ulcer Prevention Collaborative website provides information on patient safety, pressure ulcer identification and prevention in Queensland.

  —http://www.health.qld.gov.au/patientsafety/pupp/webpages/qpupc.asp

- National Guideline Clearinghouse United States provides information on various topics including pressure ulcer identification, assessment, prevention, and treatment guidelines based on pressure ulcer stage.

  —http://www.guideline.gov/summary/summary.aspx?ss=15&doc_id=11013&nbr=5793

- National Pressure Ulcer Advisory Panel Support Surface Standards Initiative.

  —http://www.npuap.org/pdf/NPUAP_S3I_TD.pdf

REFERENCES

1. Exton-Smith & Sherwin. Monitoring the mobility of patients in bed. *Medical and Biological Engineering and Computing.* Sept 1985;23(5):466–468.
2. National Pressure Ulcer Advisory Panel Support Surfaces Standards Initiative. Available at: http://www.npuap.org/pdf/ NPUAP_S3I_TD.pdf. Accessed March 10, 2008.
3. Maklebust JA, Sieggreen M. *Pressure Ulcers Guidelines for Prevention and Nursing Management.* 2nd ed. Springhouse, PA: Springhouse Corp:1996.
4. AHCPR 1992 Prevention and treatment of pressure ulcers. Pressure Ulcers in Adults: Prediction and Prevention Clinical Practice Guideline Number 3. Available online at: http://www.ncbi.nlm. nih.gov/books/bv.fcgi?rid=hstat2.chapter.4409. Accessed July 20, 2008.
5. National Pressure Ulcer Advisory Panel (NPUAP). Pressure Ulcer Stages Revised by NPUAP. Available online at www.npuap.org/ pr2.htm. Accessed June 25, 2007.
6. National Pressure Ulcer Advisory Panel (NPUAP). NPUAP Deep Tissue Injury Consensus. Available online at www.npuap.org/ DOCS/DTI.doc. Accessed June 25 2007.
7. AHCPR 1994 Treatment of pressure ulcers. Clinical Guideline Number 15. Available online at http://www.ncbi.nlm.nih.gov/ books/bv.fcgi?rid=hstat2.chapter.5124. Accessed July 20, 2008.

SUGGESTED READING

Baranoski S, Ayello E. *Wound Care Essentials Practice Principles.* Philadelphia, PA: Lippincott Williams & Wilkins; 2004.

Bryant RA. *Acute and Chronic Wounds.* 2nd ed. St. Louis, MO: Mosby; 2000.

Christian W. Standardizing the language of support surfaces. *The Remington Report.* May/June 2007:11–15.

Cuzzell J. Clues: bruised, torn skin. *AJN.* Mar 1990;93(3):16–17.

Ennis WJ, Meneses P. Wound healing at the local level: the stunned wound. *Ostomy/Wound Management.* Jan 2000;46(suppl 1A):S39–S48.

Falanga V. Wound bed preparation and the role of enzymes: a case for multiple actions of therapeutic agents. *Wounds.* 2002;14(2):47–57.

Hall JC. *Sauer's Manual of Skin Diseases*. 8th ed. Philadelphia, PA: Lippincott Williams & Wilkins; 2000.

Hess CT. *Wound Care*. 2nd ed. Springhouse, PA: Springhouse Corp; 1998.

Hess CT. *Wound Care*. 3rd ed. Springhouse, PA: Springhouse Corp; 2000.

Mertz PM, Ovington LG. Wound healing microbiology. *Dermatology Clinics*. Oct. 1993;11(4):739–747.

Papadopopoulos A, et al. Motivation and compliance in wound management. *Journal of Wound Care*. Oct 1999;8(9): 467–469.

Payne RL, et al. Defining and classifying skin tears: need for a common language. *Ostomy/Wound Management*.1993;39(5):26–37.

Petro J. Ethical and psychosocial considerations of wound management. *Decubitus*. Jan 1992;5(1):22–25.

Pettit KL, Wendt K. Across the care continuum: taking a proactive approach to pressure ulcer care. *The Remington Report*. May/June 2007;7–10.

Rhinehart E. Infection control in home care. *Emer. Infec. Dis*. 2001; 7(2):2001. *Available at: www.medscape.com*.

Rosenblum B, Harris A. Key data on pressure ulcers a cause for concern: admissions, hospitalizations, and visits on the rise. *The Remington Report*. May/June 2007:4–6.

Seidel H, Ball J, Dains J, Benedict, GW. *Mosby's Guide to Physical Examination*. 4th ed. St Louis, MO: Mosby Inc; 1999.

Stalano-Coico L, et al. Wound fluids: a reflection of the state of healing. *Ostomy/Wound Management*. Jan 2000;46(suppl 1A): S85–S93.

Sussman C, Bates-Jensen B. *Wound Care A Collaborative Practice Manual for Physical Therapists and Nurses*. Gaithersburg, MD: Aspen Publications;1998.

Support Systems International, Inc. *The Skin, Module 1*. Charleston, SC: Hillenbrand; 1993.

Swartz M. *Textbook of Physical Diagnosis History and Examination*. 3rd ed. Philadelphia, PA: W.B. Saunders; 1998.

Tierney L, McPhee S, Papadakis M. *Current Medical Diagnosis and Treatment*. 37th ed. Stamford, CT: Appleton & Lange; 1998.

White MW, et al. Skin tears in frail elders: a practical approach to prevention. *Geriatric Nursing*. 1994;15(2):95–99.

WOCN Guidance on OASIS Skin and Wound Status MO Items. Spring 2001.

Available at: http://www. deroyal.com/Wound_Care

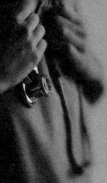

Chapter 4

LOWER EXTREMITY WOUNDS OF VENOUS INSUFFICIENCY

🔑 KEY POINTS

- Valves of the venous system are unidirectional from distal to proximal location.
- The most common cause of lower extremity ulceration is venous disease.
- Loss of valve function at differing levels results in a condition known as venous insufficiency.
- Common disease states causing valvular dysfunction include: congenital valve absence, deep vein thrombosis, phlebitis, venous hypertension, and venous engorgement.
- Venous disease may exist alone, but may also be in combination with other disease states.
- There are often characteristic skin changes, but the clinician should take a history to help in determining the type of venous disease prior to local treatment.

ETIOLOGY OF LOWER EXTREMITY WOUNDS

Some of the most challenging wounds that are seen in clinical practice are lower extremity ulcerations. It is estimated that between 70% and 90% of all leg ulcers have venous pathology.[1,2]

The most common etiology is venous insufficiency due to venous hypertension. Statistics show that in the United States 2.5 million individuals have chronic venous insufficiency (CVI) and that the chronic leg ulcers that often result affect 1.3% of the adult population.[3,4]

VENOUS SYSTEM REVIEW

The venous system mimics the arterial system; however, there is more variability anatomically than generally found in the arterial system. The veins of the leg commonly follow the tibial and peroneal arteries (Figure 4–1) and form cross-linking branches, which ascend along the artery to form the popliteal vein:

- Toward the head of the body the popliteal vein becomes the femoral vein commonly referred to as the superficial vein although it is part of the deep vein system of the leg.
- Superficial femoral vein joins the deep femoral vein forming the common femoral vein. Deep venous drainage of the leg is accomplished by the deep femoral vein.

The leg has a dual venous system, which includes the deep venous system and the superficial system. The superficial system is represented by the saphenous vein.

- Medially, the greater saphenous vein drains the leg.
- From the foot, the dorsal veins join together forming the greater saphenous vein.
- This vein is found on the medial aspect of the leg and anterior to the medial malleolus.
- Ascending the leg the greater saphenous vein becomes bifurcated and in some individuals, trifurcated.
- At the level of the knee, the greater saphenous vein becomes a deeper vein joining the common femoral.
- The lesser saphenous vein is responsible for draining the posterior aspect of the leg.
- The lesser saphenous vein merges with the popliteal vein at the calf level.
- The saphenous system connects to the deep venous system through what are known as perforator veins.
- These perforator veins shunt blood from subcutaneous tissues and the greater saphenous vein into the deep leg veins.
- Perforator veins cross through superficial fascia. Their specific location varies from individual to individual.
- The lowest perforator vein connects the entire saphenous system with the deep vein system above the medial malleolus.

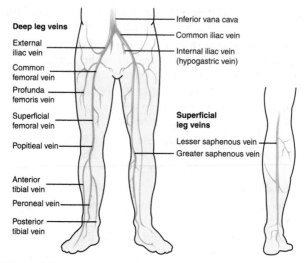

Figure 4–1 Venous system of the lower extremities. This illustration identifies the major veins in the legs from the low abdomen to the feet, and the superficial leg veins. (Reproduced with permission from Baranoski S, Ayello E. *Wound Care Essentials Practice Principles*. Philadelphia, PA: Lippincott Williams & Wilkins; 2004.)

Venous Valvular Anatomy

- The valves of the deep and superficial venous systems are located immediately before the bifurcation points in the perforator veins. These valves are unidirectional.

- These valves are oriented to shunt blood from the lesser saphenous vein and the greater saphenous system and into the deep leg veins.

- The orientation of the valves allows blood flow to proceed from a distal to proximal location.

- Each valve is a bileaflet with valve sinuses on the lateral base of each valve leaflet.

- These sinuses represent a dilation in the normal contour of the vein wall.
- Sinus function assists in valve closure, caused passively by retrograde venous blood flow into the sinus enabling the leaflets to fit together creating valve closure.
  — These leaflets are anatomically oriented parallel to the skin surface.
- Loss of valve function at differing levels results in the condition known as venous insufficiency.
- The valve leaflets become unable to fit together with overdistention of a venous segment as well as various disease states. This overdistention stretches the leaflets apart allowing blood to reflux into more dependent sections of the vein resulting in the condition known as venous insufficiency.
  — The most common disease states that may cause valvular dysfunction include:
    - Congenital valve absence
    - Deep vein thrombosis
    - Phlebitis
    - Valve atresia
    - Venous hypertension
    - Venous engorgement
- Venous blood return:
  — Smooth muscle tone of the venous walls, contraction of skeletal muscle, and negative pressure created intrathoracically during inspiration are the primary mechanisms by which venous blood is returned to the heart.
  — Hydrostatic pressure is about 90 mm Hg while standing. The pressure reaches about 120 mmHg when the calf muscle contracts during ambulation (Figure 4–2).[5]

The calf muscle pump is the most important to this function but the foot and thigh pumps also support venous return.

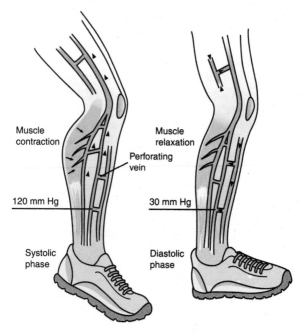

Figure 4–2 Contraction of the leg and the relaxation of the leg with movement. (Reproduced with permission from Bryant RA. *Acute and Chronic Wounds.* 2nd ed. St. Louis, MO: Mosby; 2000.)

Venous Ulcer Disease Physiology

Nursing Consideration

The most common cause of lower extremity ulceration is venous disease. The ulceration may be solely venous or may have an arterial component.

Approximately 21% of patients with venous ulcers have concomitant arterial disease.[5,6] The ulcerations result from the skin and subcutaneous tissue receiving inadequate oxygenation and nutrition due to incomplete closure of the valve. This incomplete valve closure creates a backflow of fluids which places pressure on the entire venous system in the area distal to the incompetent valve.

This is often the cause of lower extremity edema. When a patient has a venous wound, it is necessary to manage the edema for wound closure.

Etiology of Venous Hypertension

Venous stasis is no longer the current terminology; the correct terminology is venous hypertension. Prolonged venous hypertension and valvular insufficiency may be primarily in the deep vein system—femoral, popliteal, and tibial veins—or in the superficial system (greater and lesser saphenous veins or perforator veins that join the deep and superficial systems).

- Problems may exist in isolation or in combination:
- The increased venous pressure may be from conditions that create a significant disruption or impairment of the forward flow of blood, for example:
  — Chronic venous insufficiency (CVI)
  — Cardiac disease (especially Congestive Heart Failure [CHF])
  — Pelvic tumors
  — Morbid obesity
  — Increased interstitial volume (cirrhosis of liver, renal failure, protein-calorie malnutrition)
  — Result of hormone therapy

Three current pathology theories of venous hypertension are:[5,6]

- Fibrin cuff theory (from the 1980s):

  Hydrostatic pressure, venous hypertension, and venous insufficiency cause dermal ulceration over time. This is brought about by a cascade of events starting with venous hypertension leading to extravasation of fibrinogen; fibrinogen polymerizing to fibrin; to formation of fibrin cuffs which create white cell aggregation plugging the capillaries and releasing proteolytic enzymes that induce endothelial damage and further fibrinogen leakage. The fibrin cuffs impede the diffusion of oxygen and nutrients and venous ulceration occurs. This cascade of events repeats itself.

- Trap hypothesis:

    Suggests that fibrin and other macromolecules leak out through the permeable capillary beds, binding or trapping growth factors and other substances needed to maintain normal tissues and healing.[7]

- White blood cell trapping theory (currently thought to be the most accurate explanation dating from 1996–97):

    When venous hypertension exists, the blood flow from the capillaries slows down allowing leukocytes to line up, adhering to the cell walls (marginate). Some of these become trapped and plug the capillaries causing tissue ischemia. Other leukocytes migrate out into the tissues and become activated releasing proteolytic enzymes, oxygen free radicals, and other inflammatory mediators that cause tissue damage.

- Scientific evidence exists supporting the following.[7-10]

    — Transcutaneous oxygen levels are not changed when fibrin cuffs are present.

    — Venous ulcers have demonstrated healing in the presence of fibrin cuffs.

    — Fibrin cuffs may be the markers of endothelial damage, may inhibit collagen formation, and may block growth factors or other molecules necessary for healing.

    — Leukocytes marginate and some become trapped in the lower extremities of individuals with venous insufficiency.

    — Wound fluid from venous ulcers varies from that of acute wounds chemically favoring inflammation and tissue destruction.

    — Venous ulcer leakage carries a protein binding growth factors (2-macroglobulin).

NURSING ASSESSMENT

The nursing assessment includes a thorough patient history including a family history.

- Perform a thorough physical assessment.[11]

- Ask the patient about the presence of major illnesses or systemic diseases Autoimmune diseases such as rheumatoid arthritis, pyodermagranosum, or uncontrolled vasculitis will delay or inhibit wound healing.[11]
    - If the patient undergoes major surgery, wound healing is also delayed or inhibited.[11]
- Medication history[11]
    - Systemic steroids may interfere with wound healing
    - Immunosuppressive drugs will interfere with wound healing
- Nutrition assessment is also necessary as inadequate nutrition will delay or inhibit wound healing.

Observe for physical signs of the below-listed venous dysfunction risk factors and include questions about the following factors during the assessment.

Nursing Alert

A thorough review of the patient's current and recent medications is necessary. If the patient is currently taking certain medications to decrease the viscosity of the blood (e.g., Coumadin) it may preclude the use of compression therapy.

VENOUS DYSFUNCTION RISK FACTORS

- Deep venous thrombosis (DVT): may inevitably lead to ulceration, venous obstruction, and venous dilatation or varicosity; ask the patient about the presence or history of varicose veins.
    - Ask about any history of a deep vein thrombosis. The patient may identify the condition as "having had a clot in my leg."
    - If the patient has had a DVT, inquire about medications the patient is currently taking.

- Varicose veins: enlarged veins that are swollen and raised above the surface of the skin. May be dark purple or blue appearing twisted or bulging. Varicose veins are commonly found on the backs of the calves or on the medial aspect of the leg but may be in other locations as well. Varicosities develop when valves in the veins that allow blood to flow toward the heart stop working properly. This results in blood pooling in the veins and causing them to get larger. Varicose veins affect one out of two people older than 50 years and are more common in women than men.
- Hemorrhoids are a type of varicose vein.
- Spider veins are small varicose veins.
  — Always ask about patient or family history of varicose veins and deep vein thrombosis (DVT).
  — If the patient has a personal history of varicosities ask about any past treatments and their success.
- Postphlebitic syndrome
  — Always ask if the patient has a history of postphlebitic syndrome, medications taken, timeline of occurrence, and any surgical intervention.
- Congestive heart failure
  — Always ask if the patient has a history of congestive heart failure, medications taken, and weight history. Be sure to obtain a current weight to help determine treatment options.
- Incompetent valves
  — Ask if the patient has a history of incompetent valves.
- Obesity
  — Ask the patient's current weight, the most the patient has ever weighed, and ascertain current and past treatment including surgery as a treatment for obesity.
- Pregnancy
  — Ask the number of pregnancies, how many were carried to term, and if the patient used compression stockings during any or all of the pregnancies.

- Superficial vein regurgitation
  — Ask about history of superficial vein regurgitation and treatment.
- Muscle weakness secondary to paralysis and arthritis
  — The presence of weakness or arthritis may preclude the patient's ability to manage independently specific treatments such as compression stockings.
- Immobility or limited mobility with impaired calf muscle pump as in arthritis, paralysis, and muscular disorders
- Trauma
  — Crush injuries, lower leg injury, fracture, or surgery are contributing factors and potential risk factors for the development of venous insufficiency.
- Family history
  — Venous disease has strong familial predisposition.
- Cardiac disease
  — Cardiac disease (especially CHF), may be the cause of the edema.
  — CHF must be controlled while treating venous edema or venous ulcers.
- Prior venous ulcerations
  — Inquire about the location, length of time patient has been free of ulcerations, any treatment that was successful.
- Prior sores on the lower legs
  — Inquire when the patient last had such an injury, the location on his or her lower extremity, and treatment and success of treatment.

PHYSICAL CHARACTERISTICS OF VENOUS DISEASE AND VENOUS ULCERS

- Chronic dryness of the lower extremity in these patients often leads to scratching, excoriations, and eczematous changes and is referred to as 'stasis dermatitis.'

Nursing Alert
A preulcer condition is often misdiagnosed as cellulitus and is characterized by lower extremity edema, induration, and erythematous hyperpigmentation of the leg.

- Usually occurs in the gaiter area—medial aspect of the lower leg—often just proximal and superior to the medial malleolus or great saphenous vein location
- Large in size although may start small
- Wound edges are diffuse, flat, and sloping although the wound is usually shallow and may be beefy red in color
- Exudate from wound bed is common and may be serous, serosanguinous, yellow, or other colors
- Generalized edema is common and if the edema is not controlled, blisters may occur and progress to open ulcerations
- Hyperpigmentation or hemosiderin pigmentation—brownish staining—is nearly always present
  - Hemosiderin staining is a yellow-brown, granular, iron-containing pigment derived from the breakdown of hemoglobin. Hemosiderosis is a brown or rusty discoloration of the skin resulting from a buildup of hemosiderin in the interstitial fluid. Hemosiderin staining is an outcome of venous hypertension, where there is extravasation of red blood cells into the tissues. Over time these red blood cells (and their hemoglobin) begin to break down and hemosiderin deposits result.[7]
- Pain may be significant; often a dull aching sensation, heaviness of extremity, and typically increases during the day with prolonged limb dependency
  - May be alleviated with limb elevation.
  - Some individuals experience sudden "bursting" pain also known as venous claudication, caused by venous congestion in response to increased blood flow during exercise. This may be misinterpreted as intermittent claudication of ischemic disease.

— May worsen in warm weather, humid weather.

— May worsen during menses.

— Generally worsens with sodium and water retention due to increased edema.

• Scaly, itching dermatitis is usually present with exfoliation

— May be due to either endogenous or exogenous factors.

— Severe allergic reactions may complicate the plan of care (POC).

— Chemical or mechanical factors are most often the cause of contact dermatitis around a leg ulcer—often referred to as the periwound skin.

• Pulses are present and usually palpable after edema is managed; remember that approximately 20% of patients may have an anatomical anomaly and may not have a pedal pulse

---

 Nursing Alert

It is important to rule out gross arterial disease by physical examination and ankle brachial index (ABI).[11] Remember that if the patient has mixed disease (venous and arterial disease), treating only the venous disease is not sufficient.

• Yellow, gelatinous fibrin commonly accumulates in the ulcer.

• Dilated superficial veins are commonly called telangiectasias or spider veins.

• In advanced disease the thick, tender, indurated, and fibrosed commonly dermal and subcutaneous tissue of liposclerosis may be seen; this often occurs before the ulceration.

• White, avascular, sclerotic areas known as Atrophie blanche are another potential finding.

— Refers to smooth, ivory-white plaques in the skin. These plaques are avascular (having few or no blood vessels), sclerotic (hardened) areas that are prone to ulcer formation due to the relative lack of oxygen and nutrient flow to the area.[12]

— Capillaroscopic studies have shown dense loops of glomerulus-like capillaries with microvascular obstructions.

• These ulcers often develop slowly and can exist for years.

PHYSICAL ASSESSMENT OF THE EXTREMITY

Assessment of the lower extremity includes evaluating the presence or absence of pulses (Table 4–1) and the absence or presence of edema (Figure 4–3).

• To assess pitting edema, press your index finger over the bony prominence of the tibia or medial malleolus for several seconds. A depression that does not rapidly refill and resume its original contour indicates orthostatic (pitting) edema, which is not usually accompanied by thickening or pigmentation of the overlying skin.

— 1+: slight pitting; no visible distortion; disappears rapidly

— 2+: a somewhat deeper pit than in 1+, but again no readily detectable distortion; disappears in 10 to 15 seconds

— 3+: the pit is noticeably deep; may last more than 1 minute; the dependent extremity looks fuller and swollen

Table 4–1 Grading of Pulses

Pulses	
0	Absent
1+	Barely palpable
2+	Palpable but diminished
3+	Normal
4+	Prominent, suggestive of an aneurysm

From: Hallett JW, et al. *Manual of Patient Care in Vascular Surgery*. Boston, MA: Little, Brown & Co; 1982.

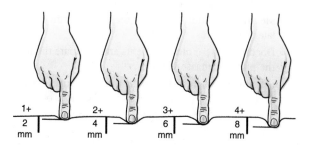

Figure 4–3 Assessing pitting edema. (Reproduced with permission from Seidel H, Ball J, Dains J, Williams BG: *Mosby's Guide to Physical Examination.* 4th ed. St. Louis, MO: Mosby; 1999.)

— 4+: the pit is very deep; lasts as long as 2 to 5 minutes; the dependent extremity is grossly distorted

— If edema is unilateral, suspect the occlusion of a major vein. If edema occurs without pitting, suspect arterial disease and occlusion.[12]

MANAGEMENT OF LOWER EXTREMITY WOUNDS AND EDEMA

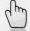 **Nursing Alert**
Edema must be controlled to adequately manage the wound.

- Quantitative measures: document the following quantitative measures to compare current outcomes with past measurements to determine the efficacy of treatment

  — Leg circumference: measure with an individual disposable tape

    ■ Measure the calf 10 centimeters below the inferior rim of the patella at the visually largest area

- Measure 5 centimeters above the superior rim of the lateral malleolus
- Document these measurements and compare them to the previous measurements
— Qualitative measures: document the qualitative measures and compare current observations with previous outcomes.
  - Appearance of the lower extremity in general
  - Shininess of the skin
  - Exudate amount, color, odor, and consistency
  - Patient's sense of weight or heaviness of the limb
  - If compression wraps are used, evaluate for areas of ridging or bulging between folds of the wrap
  - Evaluate for bulging above or below the compression wrap
  - Evaluate for wounds above or below the compression wrap
  - Ask the patient if edema subsides overnight with leg elevation
  - Ask patient about his or her use of foot gear and clothing

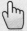

Nursing Tip
It is important to the POC and planned outcomes for the patient to:
— Wear clothing that is lightweight and does not bind or constrict arterial or venous blood flow.
— Wear foot gear that does not bind or constrict the foot or ankle. The sole should be relatively flat (no high heels). It is often advisable where possible for the patient to wear shoes that can be laundered or cleaned in the case of excess fluid staining the foot gear. Ask the patient if edema subsides over night with leg elevation.

TREATMENT OF VENOUS ULCERS

- Assess at each visit the patient's participation and perceptions about the treatment regimen. The patient's understanding and expectations for success should be evaluated and discussed. Many lower extremity ulcers may heal very slowly and require a long duration of treatment.

- Dermatitis requires treatment often with a steroid. These medications can often only be used for 14 days at a time or if atrophy of the skin occurs. Consult with a physician.

- Repetitive episodes of infection and cellulitis require treatment as they may cause lymphatic system damage and lymphedema. Consult with a physician.

- Loss of ankle function may occur due to fibrosis and bony ankylosis.

- Educate patients regarding ankle pump exercises using clockwise and counterclockwise circles.

- Encourage ambulation to tolerance several times every day.

- Cellulitus must be treated. A culture and systemic treatment may be necessary. Consult with a physician.

- Edema must be relieved for wounds to heal.

- Patient's legs should be elevated above heart level WITHOUT compression on the femoral arteries and limited or reduced pressure on the sacrum, coccyx, and ischial tuberosities.

- Leg elevation must be performed every day for at least double the time the leg is dependent.

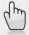

Nursing Tip
Remember to have the patient utilize pressure reduction devices when elevating the legs. These devices include mattresses, overlays, chair pads, and pressure reduction boots for the legs and heels.

- Some studies indicate that diuretic therapy used to control venous edema may cause cellular changes in the skin of the lower legs that actually retards healing.[2]

Compression Therapy

Compression therapy is NOT the use of elastic wraps. It is the use of medical grade compression garments or devices. For example, ace wraps or other athletic/sports wraps.

Nursing Precaution

Use compression therapy only if palpable pulses (dorsalis pedis and post tibial) are readily detected. If not, refer the patient to the attending physician for vascular studies.

- It is helpful to obtain ankle-arm indexes (AAIs) on the patient before determining the type and amount of compression to be used.
  - This must be no less than 0.8 for compression therapy; also known as ankle-brachial indexes (ABIs)
  - Remember to treat any dermatitis that may be present
  - Remember to treat the scaly, exfoliation even if there is no dermatitis
    - Any lotion or cream is appropriate; however, inquire about patient allergies before application.
- Compression therapy types include:
  - Graduated compression stockings
    - Light support
      - 8 to 14 mmHG; fashion hosiery (Jobst, Sigvarus, Juzo)
      - Used primarily for edema prevention in individuals who require standing or sitting without much activity; mild, early varicose veins.
      - Class 1: 14 to 18 mmHg compression
- Antiembolism stockings
  - 16 to 18 mm Hg, Jobst, TED
  - Used for deep vein thrombosis (DVT) prophylaxis in non-ambulatory edematous patients. Not recommended for edema control in the ambulatory patient.

- Low compression stockings
  - Class 2: 18 to 24 mmHg, Relief (Jobst), elastic wraps, paste bandages provide medium compression.
  - Used in edematous, nonambulatory patients when antiembolism stockings have failed; acute DVT, treatment and prevention of venous ulceration.
- Low to moderate compression stockings and wraps
  - Class 3: 25 to 35 mmHg, Fast-Fit (Jobst), Custom Fit, double reverse elastic wrap, four-layer bandage.
  - Used when edema is secondary to venous insufficiency; severe chronic venous hypertension, severe varicose veins, ulcer prevention and treatment in patients with very large diameter calves.
  - Patient participates in exercise rehabilitation while wearing the stockings.
- Moderate compression stockings and wraps
  - 30 to 40 mmHg, Ultimate (Jobst), Custom stocking (Jobst, Sigvarus), Sequential pump, four-layer bandage (Profore, Smith & Nephew or SurePress, Convatec-Squibb)
  - Used for the patient with or without wounding, persistent edema despite lower level compression options, or in the ulcer that failed to heal after 6 months.
- High compression stockings and devices
  - 30 to 40 mmHg, Vairox (Jobst), Custom stockings (Jobst, Sigvarus), Sequential pump
  - Used with lymphedema patients
  - Class 4: 40 to 50 mmHg compression
- General information on compression garments and stockings:
  - Usually wounds must be healed before using stockings.
  - Wound must be healed to 1 cm length by 1 cm width by 1 cm shallow depth; compression hosiery (30–40 mmHg) or milder compression (10–30 mmHg) may be appropriate to use after other forms of compression have been used successfully.

— Stockings are a prescription item and the patient must be measured for them.

— Antiembolic stockings are not indicated for compression therapy. Generally, below-knee stockings are sufficient.

▪ Patients with severe postphlebitic syndrome or lymphedema may require thigh-high stockings but may need to have a vascular physician evaluate and prescribe the stockings.

• Level of compression:

— Patient should be encouraged to purchase two pair of stockings at a time so one can be worn while the other is washed and dried.

— Stockings should be refitted and replaced every 6 months and in most cases, the patients will need to wear them for life.

— Stockings are often difficult to apply for patients with arthritis and others with arm or hand conditions. An evaluation from occupational therapy is needed to provide adaptive devices for activities of daily living (ADLs).

• Continuous wrap (noncompression) (Figure 4–4)

• Example is Unna's boot

— Impregnated with moist paste usually consisting of zinc oxide, gelatin, and glycerin (some contain calamine).

— Applied in a circular fashion from the foot to just below the patella upon awakening in the morning; however, it is always important to verify the patient's schedule and habits.

— Applied without tension when edema has subsided; should be covered with a gauze to protect clothing.

— These dressings do NOT provide compression but many of the various brands dry and stiffen with age. When this occurs the leg cannot swell inside the wrap but may swell above and below the wrap.

— A compression wrap may be placed over the Unna's boot to enhance compression.

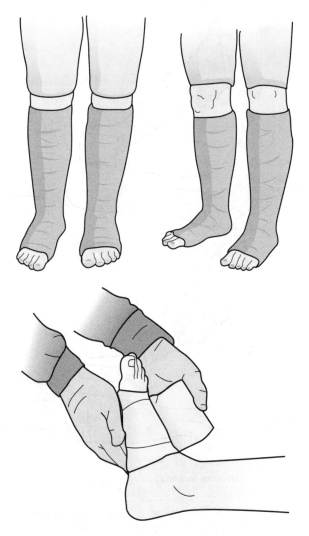

Figure 4–4 Extremity in a wrap. (*Continued*)

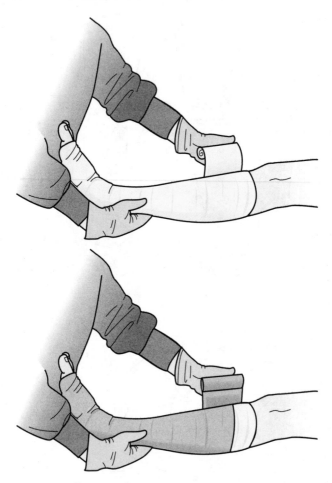

Figure 4–4 Extremity in a wrap.

— The use of a compression covering such as Coban may also be used and does apply some compression.
— The wrap must be applied from the toes to the infrapatellar notch (this is the area of least compression).

- Continuous compression via compression wrap
  — Provides graduated, sustained compression.
  — Some of these are layered dressings such as Profore, a four-layered wrap that includes both circular wrapping and figure-8 wrapping.
    - Four layers include protection, padding, and compression.
    - Most wraps are left in place for 3 to 7 days while a wound is present.

Nursing Consideration

Various dressing types may be used under compression wraps if infection in the wound is NOT present. These wraps are usually occlusive in nature and are not meant for use until an infection is controlled. Remember that improper wrapping technique may cause cellulitus.

- Compression via tubular, shaped, elasticized bandages
  — A dressing is applied with a tubular bandage over this (Tubigrip, Setopress).
  — Slightly increases the compression; may reduce dressing slippage.
  — Useful with patients who cannot tolerate an elastic compression bandage.
  — Intermittent compression via wraps that are applied once each day and removed at night.
- Sequential via pneumatic compression device
  — Patient should elevate the legs for 30 minutes before applying the pump.
  — Pumping is done twice a day for 2 hours at a time and works well when the patient is able to adhere to the treatment regimen.

Nursing Tips

Choose the compression type carefully.

- Explain and educate the patient regarding the rationale for use.
- Assist the patient with weight loss.
- Assist the patient with adherence to the regimen.

- Provide thorough, easily understandable written instructions with diagrams or pictures.
- Instruct the patient to follow up with a health-care professional on a routine basis.
- If the wounds demonstrate regression or do not demonstrate progression, evaluate the entire treatment regimen and make appropriate changes.
- Encourage the patient to ambulate to tolerance while using all compression garments, stockings, compression wraps, and Unna's boot.
- Wraps are not intended to be kept in place when the patient is confined to bed.
- Include a leg exercise program and elevation as an essential part of the POC in all patients with venous insufficiency (see Tables 4–2 and 4–3).
- Leg Exercise and elevation
  — Frequency: 20 to 30 minutes every 2 to 3 hours while awake for total of at least 2 to 4 hours every day.
  — Elevate the foot of the bed while sleeping using 4-inch blocks.
- Expected outcomes of leg exercise and elevation: lower extremity edema and discomfort is reduced or eliminated.

Table 4–2 Leg Exercise and Elevation

Indications	Contraindications
Lower extremity edema secondary to venous return impairment	Morbid obesity
	Arterial occlusive disease and ischemic pain with elevation
	CHF limits ability to recline
	Other medical conditions limiting or prohibiting reclining

Table 4–3   Leg Exercise and Elevation

Advantages	Disadvantages
No financial cost	Consistent performance for benefits
Effective with regular use in combination with treatments	Patient unable to elevate legs higher than heart
No special equipment required	Setting not conducive to reclining or elevation
	Ineffective in some forms of edema

- Compression wraps (elastic bandages) (Tables 4–4 and 4–5)
  - A short stretch elastic bandage that causes movement of excess fluid from the extremity when applied to the leg.
  - Frequency: wrap area within 20 minutes of rising; reapplication of wrap telescopes or slides down the leg.
- Remove at bedtime (hs).
- Expected outcomes
  - Lower extremity edema is eliminated or decreased. Results documented as a decrease in calf and ankle circumference.
  - Patient or caregiver is independent in wrapping the area, managing edema, and maintaining a weight log.

Table 4–4   Indications and Contraindications of Compression Wraps

Indications	Contraindications
Lower extremity edema secondary to impaired venous return	ABI less than 0.8
Edema reduction prior to compression stocking fitting	Patient or caregiver unable to apply bandages
Patient or caregiver able to apply elastic bandages	Allergy or sensitivity to any components such as latex

Table 4–5 Advantages and Disadvantages of Compression Wraps

Advantages	Disadvantages
Inexpensive	Practice makes perfect
Readily available	Uneven tension if not careful
Easily removed	Telescoping or sliding down leg
Active participation of patient and caregiver	Patient or caregiver unable to reach toes to wrap from foot to knee
	Requires patient or caregiver commitment to wearing for benefits

- Paste bandage (Tables 4–6 and 4–7)
  — Should be applied when the limb is without edema.
  — As it dries the paste bandage resists additional swelling.
  — Apply every 3 to 7 days but more frequently if heavy exudate is not contained.
  — MUST be changed immediately if the patient or caregiver notices excessive exudate, foul odor, or severe pain.

Table 4–6 Indications and Contraindications of Paste Bandages

Indications	Contraindications
Patient or caregiver unable to adhere to other treatments for edema control	Patient or caregiver has poor personal hygiene
Patient or caregiver unable to wrap legs daily and independently	ABI less than 0.8
Patient awaiting custom compression garment for interval edema control	Frail, friable skin of lower extremity
	Active cellulitus
	Lower extremity infected wounds

Table 4–7 **Advantages and Disadvantages of Paste Bandages**

Advantages	Disadvantages
Useful when patient or caregiver unable to adhere to other treatments for edema control	Patient unable to shower or tub bathe with bandage in place
Useful when patient or caregiver unable to contribute to self-care	Unless patient or caregiver is applying the dressing, ownership of the problem is transferred to health-care system or provider
Eliminates or decreases daily dressing changes	Odor when time to change bandage
	New ulcerations with improper wrapping

- Expected outcomes
    - Wrap remains in place for 7 days after application.
    - Lower extremity edema is controlled
    - Measurements of ankle and calf circumference decrease
- Additional information on paste bandages
- Patient may remove wrap before provider visit to shower (no tub baths or soaking) if legs are elevated when more than 20 minutes will elapse from the time of removal to replacement.
- Read the directions as some of these wraps require a figure-8 method for application while others require a circular application.
- Cotton padding (i.e., cast padding) may be used for excessive exudate absorption if placed at skin level.
- If the wrap becomes uncomfortable or too tight after the patient has been up and active, the patient should elevate the lower extremities above heart level for 30 minutes. If discomfort is relieved, the patient may resume activities; if no relief, the patient should either be seen by a health-care professional or remove the wrap until he or she is able to consult with a health-care professional.

Table 4–8   Indications and Contraindications of Four-Layer Bandages

Indications	Contraindications
Patient or caregiver unable to adhere to other treatment for edema control	Patient or caregiver has poor personal hygiene
Patient or caregiver unable to independently wrap lower extremity daily	Patient has significant arterial occlusive disease, ABI less than 0.8
Patient awaiting custom garment	Active cellulitis
	Lower extremity infected wounds

- During application the wrap should be cut to avoid pleats, folds, or wrinkles that may cause damage to the skin.
- Use calamine-free wraps in patients allergic or sensitive to calamine. Evaluate before wrapping.
- Patients with inverted champagne bottle leg—narrow ankle and large calf—will most likely need ankle padding with dressings (e.g., ABD pad) or cotton cast material to avoid overpressurizing the calf.
- Four-Layer bandage (Tables 4–8 and 4–9)
  - If applied correctly, this system provides 40 mmHg ankle pressure graduating to 17 mmHg at the calf.
  - Apply every 4 to 7 days or more frequently if excessive exudate is present.
  - Change immediately if the patient experiences severe pain, excessive exudate, or foul odor.
- Expected outcomes
  - Wrap remains in place for 7 days
  - Lower extremity edema is controlled
  - Measurements of ankle and calf circumference are decreased
- Additional information on four-layer bandages

Table 4–9   Advantages and Disadvantages of Four-Layer
Bandages

Advantages	Disadvantages
Useful with patient or care-giver unable to adhere to other treatments for edema control.	Patient unable to shower or bathe while bandage in place.
Useful with patient or caregiver unable to contribute to self-care.	Unless patient or caregiver doing application, ownership of the problem is transferred to the health-care system or provider. Uncommon for patient or caregiver to be taught this dressing technique.
Decreases or eliminates daily dressing changes.	Odor when time to change bandage.
	New ulcerations can occur with improper wrapping.

— Patient may remove bandage before provider visit to shower (no tub baths or soaking) if legs are elevated when more than 20 minutes will elapse from the time of removal to replacement.

— If the wrap becomes uncomfortable or too tight after the patient has been up and active, the patient should elevate the lower extremities above heart level for 30 minutes. If discomfort is relieved, the patient may resume activities; if no relief, the patient should either be seen by a health-care professional or remove the wrap until he or she is able to consult with a health-care professional.

— Patient with inverted champagne bottle leg will most likely need ankle padding with dressings (e.g., ABD pad) or cotton cast material to avoid overpressurizing the calf.

— Some wraps require a certain ankle circumference before the wrap is applied. Most are not to be used on patients with diabetes mellitus.

Table 4-10   Indications and Contraindications of Compression
Stockings and Garments

Indications	Contraindications
Venous disease	Patient has significant arterial occlusive disease, ABI less than 0.8
Lymphedema	Allergy or sensitivity to components such as latex

- Compression stockings and garments (Tables 4-10 and 4-11)
  — Measured and fitted to the patient for the provision of external compression of the extremity at prescribed levels.
  — Garments are available for many body parts such as the upper and lower extremities including knee high, thigh high, and waist high.
  — Garment should be applied before getting out of bed for the day and removed immediately before retiring.
  — Stockings are available in various colors and materials including cotton.
  — Manufacturer's instructions concerning care must be followed.

Table 4-11   Advantages and Disadvantages of Compression
Stockings and Garments

Advantages	Disadvantages
Graded compression	Difficult to put on for some patients and caregivers.
Many last 4-9 months (manufacturer dependent)	Cost not always insurance covered. Custom garments are usually expensive.
Various types	Patient and caregiver must be committed to patient's wearing garment.
Cosmetically acceptable	NOT for patients with extensive leg wounds or circumferential wounds.

— Stocking "butlers," donners, or aids are available and assist patients and caregivers in placing the stockings.
- Expected outcomes
  — Patient or caregiver is able to apply garment with minimal difficulty.
  — Garment is on the patient when the health-care provider arrives for visit.
  — Lower extremity edema is controlled.
  — Measurements of ankle and calf circumference are decreased and clinical improvement is noted.

Nursing Consideration

The patient should be measured for the garment at the time of day when there is the least amount of swelling; may need to use the sequential pump for 1 to 2 hours before the fitting appointment.

Nursing Tip
For patients who cannot or will not utilize adequate compression garments, intermittent pneumatic pressure (IPC) is an option.[11]

TREATMENT OF DERMATITIS

- Determine the underlying cause.
- Treat with corticosteroid ointment (fewer preservatives than creams/lotions).
- Betamethasone dipropionate ointment (Diprolene); potency Group 1 is the most potent; also available in Group 2 strength. Consult with physician for treatment.
- Triamcinolone acetonide ointment (Aristocort) or Fluocinolone acetonide ointment (Synalar); potency Group 4. Consult with physician for treatment.

- Treatment for 7 to 14 days; then discontinue to avoid skin side effects.
- Newer silver dressings may also have a role in topical management of venous ulcers in the presence of local infection.
- Newer biological dressings such as skin replacement may also have a role in topical management. These dressings often (except OASIS Healthpoint) may require application by a physician, physician assistant, or nurse practitioner.

 Nursing Tip

AVOID occlusive dressings and wraps if cellulitis is present. Alleviate this condition first with oral or intravenous antibiotics.

INTERNET RESOURCES

The following websites provide patient and health-care provider information, graphics, and handouts.

- **New York University Medical Center and School of Medicine website has English and Spanish language patient education materials, health-care provider information.**

  —http://www.med.nyu.edu/patientcare/library/article.html? ChunkIID=22580
- **Adventist Health Care website has patient and health-care provider information.**

  —http://www.adventisthealthcare.com/AHC/health/library/ Health_Illustrated_Encyclopedia/1/1_000203.aspx

REFERENCES

1. Lopez AP, et al. Venous Ulcers. *Wounds*. 1998;10(5):149.
2. Reichardt LE. Venous Ulceration:compression as the mainstay of therapy. *JWOCN*. 1999;26(1):39.

3. Mozes G, et al. A Surgical Anatomy for Endoscopic Subfascial Division of Perforating Veins. *Journal of Vascular Surgery.* 1996;24:800–808.

4. Queral LA, et al. Mini-incisional ligation of incompetent perforating veins of the legs. *Journal of Vascular Surgery.* 1997;25:437–441.

5. O'Donnell TF, et al. Chronic Venous Insufficiency. In: Jarrett F et al. *Vascular Surgery of the Lower Extremities.* St. Louis, MO: Mosby;1996.

6. O'Donnell TF, et al. Chronic venous insuffiency and varicose veins. In: Young, JR et al. *Peripheral Vascular Diseases,* 2nd ed. St. Louis, MO: Mosby; 1996.

7. Falanga V. Wound Bed Preparation and the Role of Enzymes: A Case for Multiple Actions of Therapeutic Agents. *Wounds.* 2002;14(2): 47–57.

8. Venous Definations. Available at: http://www.seniors.gov.ab.ca/AADL/AV/manual/PDF/44b_venous_definitions.pdf. Accessed July 7, 2007.

9. Hallett JW et al. *Manual of Patient Care in Vascular Surgery.* Boston, MA: Little, Brown & Co; 1982.

10. Bergan JJ, Schmid-Schönbein GW, Smith PDC, Nicolaides AN; Boisseau MR, Eklof B. Mechanisms of disease: chronic venous disease. *New England Journal of Medicine.* Aug 2006;355(5): 488–98, 539.

11. Robson MC, et al. Guidelines for the treatment of venous ulcers. *Wound Repair and Regeneration.* 2006;14:649–662.

12. Varicose Veins. Available at: http://www.nlm.nih.gov/medlineplus/varicoseveins.html. Accessed July 04, 2007.

SUGGESTED READING

Baranoski S, Ayello E. *Wound Care Essentials Practice Principles.* Philadelphia, PA: Lippincott Williams & Wilkins; 2004.

Bryant RA. *Acute and Chronic Wounds.* 2nd ed. St. Louis, MO: Mosby; 2000.

Hampton S. An introduction to various types of leg ulcers and their management. *British Journal of Nursing.* June 2006;15(suppl): S9–S10, S12–S13.

Seaman S. Evaluation and management of lower extremity ulcers: adherence to prescribed therapy can save limbs. *Advance for Nurse Practitioners*. Mar 2002;10(3):32–47.

Seidel H, Ball J, Dains J, Benedict GW. *Mosby's Guide to Physical Examination*. 4th ed. St. Louis, MO: Mosby; 1999.

Sussman C, Bates-Jensen B. *Wound Care, A Collaborative Practice Manual for Physical Therapists and Nurses*. Gaithersburg, MD: Aspen Publications; 1998.

Worley CA. 'It hurts when I walk:' venous stasis disease—differential diagnosis and treatment. *Dermatology Nursing*. Dec 2006;18(6): 582–3.

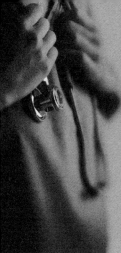

Chapter 5

ARTERIAL INSUFFICIENCY, ULCER ASSESSMENT, AND MANAGEMENT PRINCIPLES

KEY POINTS

- Facts of PAOD
- Pathophysiology of PAOD
- Risk factors and arterial ulcer characteristics

KEY DEFINITIONS

Amputation: complete or partial removal of a limb or body appendage by surgical or traumatic means.

Gangrene: the death or necrosis of a part of the body secondary to injury, infection, and/or lack of blood supply. This indicates irreversible damage where healing cannot be anticipated without loss of some part of the extremity.

Ischemia: the impairment of blood flow secondary to an obstruction of constriction of arterial flow.

Neuropathy: nerve dysfunction affecting sensory, motor, and/or autonomic fibers with varying degrees of impairment, symptoms, and signs. Diabetic peripheral neuropathy is the presence of symptoms and/or of signs of peripheral nerve dysfunction in people with diabetes after exclusion of other causes.

Ulceration: a partial or full thickness defect in the skin that may extend to subcuticular tissue, tendon, muscle, bone, or joint.

PERIPHERAL VASCULAR DISEASE FACTS

The etiology of arterial ulcers is often labeled "peripheral vascular disease" or PVD. This term actually includes venous and lymphatic system conditions and diseases; therefore, it is important for the health-care provider to consider the entire spectrum when a patient presents with a lower extremity wound. PAOD is the abbreviation for "peripheral arterial occlusive disease."

- PAOD
  - Affects approximately 10 million individuals in the United States[2]
  - Increases with age

— Affects more men than women[2]

— Clinically significant (symptomatic) disease in less than 2% of men 50 years and younger; it increases to 5% to 6% in men 70 years and older[4]

- The disease follows the same pattern in women but with a 10-year delay; reaches 5% to 6% of women at 80 years[2]

  — Asymptomatic disease in 19% of those 55 years and older[3]

  — Arterial ulceration is uncommon even with symptomatic PAOD.

  — Severe ischemia (intermittent claudication) develops in less than 25% of those with symptomatic arterial insufficiency[5]

  — Approximately 3% to 5% will require amputation due to PAOD and its complications[3]

- The outcome for an individual diagnosed with severe ischemia is poor unless aggressive intervention targeted at interrupting or reversing the pathologic process is employed in a timely manner.

  — Severe ischemia is associated with an annual mortality rate of 20%.[3]

  — Of these deaths, 50% are caused by coronary artery disease.[5,3]

- In the United States, chronic venous disease is the seventh most common chronic disease causing 70% to 90% of all leg ulcers. Therefore, the majority of leg ulcers in the United States are of venous etiology.[5]

  — Unlike PAOD, the majority of individuals with venous ulcers are female.

  — Approximately 3.5% of these women are older than 65 years.[5]

  — Studies indicate that venous ulcers have a significant impact on the life of those individuals with this condition.

- Chronic pain and discomfort create social isolation, inability to work, and feelings of anger and resentment.
- Frequent hospitalizations and clinic visits for care affect lifestyle.
- Additionally, over 2 million work days are lost each year in the United States as a result of postphlebitic syndrome.[5]

— Similar studies among individuals with PAOD have not been done; however, peripheral arterial disease, arterial insufficiency, and arterial ulcers also result in lifestyle changes. Therefore, similar psychological, sociological, and financial conditions are the most likely outcomes.

REVIEW OF THE ARTERIAL SYSTEM

- Arterial flow moves from the heart downward (Figure 5–1).
- Lower extremity arterial perfusion is initiated with satisfactory cardiac performance.
  — First arterial collateral vessels of importance to leg perfusion are the intercostal arteries arising from the descending thoracic aorta.
  — They are the only collaterals in distal aortic occlusion.
- The greatest reduction in size of the aorta occurs distal to the renal arteries.
  — Lumbar arteries are usually paired vessels at each vertebral level in the abdomen and are important to lower extremities as collateral pathways when the patient has severe aorto-iliac occlusive disease or distal aortic occlusions.
  — Internal iliac arteries through the gluteal and pudental branches are another collateral pathway to leg perfusion.
  — The external iliac artery at the level of the inguinal ligament becomes the common femoral artery. This vessel bifurcates into the deep femoral and superficial femoral arteries.

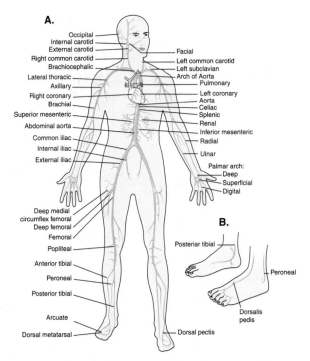

Figure 5–1 The arterial system. *A*, Arterial structure of lower extremity. *B*, Peroneal artery, posterior tibialis, and dorsalis pedis. (Reprinted with permission from Bryant RA. *Acute and Chronic Wounds*. 2nd ed. 2000.)

- Most important collateral pathway for perfusion of the lower leg is the deep femoral artery with its muscular perforators.
  — In those individuals with peripheral occlusive disease, the superficial femoral artery is the most often occluded artery resulting in ischemia of the lower leg.
  — The superficial femoral artery becomes the popliteal artery after exiting the adductor hiatus. This artery bifurcates into the tibioperoneal trunk and the anterior tibial artery.

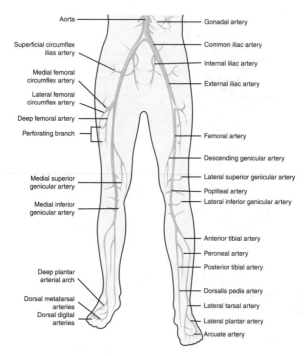

Figure 5–1 (C) Arterial Structure of Lower Extremity.
(Reproduced with permission from *Wound Care Made Incredibly Easy*. 2nd ed. Philadelphia, PA: Lippincott Williams and Wilkins; 2007.)

— The peroneal artery descends toward the ankle through deep musculature while the posterior tibial descends more superficially into the foot.

  ▪ The peroneal artery is most often patent even in individuals with severe lower extremity peripheral vascular occlusive disease.

— The anterior and posterior tibial arteries descend into the foot. The palpable anterior tibial artery becomes the dorsalis pedis artery while the posterior tibial artery provides deep and superficial components of the plantar arch.

- Perforators of the plantar arch provide arterial perfusion to the heel, sole of the foot, and branch into the digits.
- The anterior tibial artery communicates with the plantar arch, which completes the circulation of the foot.
- The peroneal artery provides perfusion to the medial and lateral tarsal branches, which communicate with the more distal aspects of the anterior and posterior tibial arteries.
- Bypass operations may be to any of these vessels.

Arterial Anatomy and Physiology

- Arterial anatomy and physiology (Figure 5–2A).
- Arteries are more muscular than veins, and those vessels located below the common femoral artery are able to adjust more rapidly in size relative to perfusion.
  — Tibioperoeal arteries rapidly accommodate perfusion changes by either relaxing or dilating.
- When atherosclerotic (plaque formation) accumulation decreases the interior size of the vessel, arteries are able to increase in size to maintain a constant shear stress until the stenosis in the vessel reaches approximately 50% of its diameter. At this point, the artery is unable to relax any further and an increase in plaque formation will impede perfusion. Continued stenosis from plaque will decrease the diameter of the artery distal to the stenosis to accommodate reduced blood flow (Figure 5–2B).
- Calcific atherosclerosis will cause the arterial wall to become more rigid.
- Perfusion in the arteries:
  — The more slowly blood flows through an artery the more viscous the blood becomes. This is also known as shear rate or velocity of blood flow.
    - Hematocrit is the more important determinant of whole blood viscosity; therefore, as red blood cell mass increases so does the viscosity.

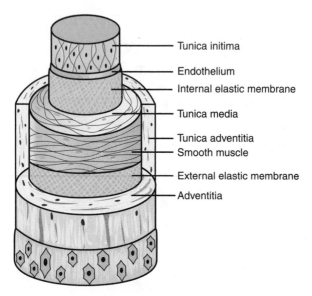

Figure 5–2A Anatomy of a Blood Vessel. (Reproduced with permission from *Wound Care Made Incredibly Easy.* 2nd ed. Philadelphia, PA: Lippincott Williams and Wilkins; 2007.)

- Conditions that contribute to the increase in viscosity are dehydration and polycythemia. Mild dehydration in an older individual may result in a decrease of extremity perfusion. Rehydrating an elderly person may therefore reduce the red cell mass and allow improved perfusion

- In the case of abnormal concentrations of proteins such as multiple myeloma, which increases viscosity, the treatment of choice may be plasmapheresis.

— Another determinant of perfusion is red blood cell (RBC) deformity or how readily the individual RBCs change cell shape. If the individual has a condition that causes the RBCs to maintain rigid cell membranes, tissue perfusion decreases from the precapillary to postcapillary level.

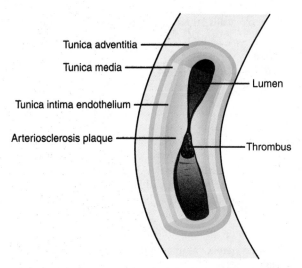

Figure 5–2B Stenosis created by plaque. (Reproduced with permission from *Wound Care Made Incredibly Easy*. 2nd ed. Philadelphia, PA: Lippincott Williams and Wilkins; 2007.)

- Pentoxifylline (Trental) may enable the RBC to more readily deform thereby increasing perfusion of the tissues.
- Muscle tissue is also able to change its metabolic requirements, becoming more efficient under anaerobic conditions such as long distance running. Although this is a gradual process, it is useful in the treatment of claudication.
  - Regular exercise can increase the distance walked before pain from claudication occurs.

Pathophysiology of Arterial Disease

Categorization of arterial disease is commonly based on the anatomical location of the problem. The condition is caused by total or partial occlusion of some portion of the arterial system such as bowel necrosis, brain attack or stroke, or arterial leg ulcer.

Morphologically, there are four classifications of arterial lesions:

1. Obstruction
2. Disruption (trauma induced)
3. Fistula
4. Dilatation (aneurysm)

The first three classifications may be responsible for causing tissue necrosis. Ulcerations are usually due to poor tissue perfusion from arterial insufficiency secondary to peripheral vascular disease, cardiovascular disease, or diabetes mellitus. The disease may be acute or chronic in nature and based on the location of resultant damage, may be classified as either organic or functional.

Functional damage:

- Causes reversible vasomotor disturbance such as Raynaud's disease.
- Affects the upper extremities causing pain and pallor but rarely ischemic necrosis.
- Causes development of dilated capillaries and venules resulting in purplish discolored areas that become ulcerations also known as *Livedo reticularis*.

Organic damage:

- Causes structural changes in the artery wall or the lumen obstructing blood flow.
- Arteriosclerosis obliterans (ASO) is the most frequent and significant organic disease in ulcer development.
  - The etiology is almost always atherosclerosis—an accumulation of cells, debris, fibers, and lipids in the intimal wall of the vessel resulting in chronic, progressive hardening and occlusion of the arteries
  - Causes a narrowing of the arterial vessel lumen and therefore obstructs arterial blood flow (50% reduction of arterial diameter on arteriogram correlates with 75% stenosis of cross-section of vessel).

- Most common locations of occlusion are the areas of bifurcation in the pelvis and lower extremities (Figure 5–3).
— Progresses over years, and blood flow is unaffected until a cross-sectional area of the artery is reduced by about 75%.
— The body develops collateral circulation in an attempt to compensate for the obstruction and thereby maintaining circulatory viability of the affected area. When the collateral circulation is unable to provide enough blood flow for exercising muscles intermittent claudication results. The primary symptom of this is crampy pain in the lower extremities occurring with exercise. This is most common in the buttocks, thighs, and calf muscles regardless of which proximal artery is obstructed. These arteries have a great demand for oxygen from the blood.
  - The pain disappears with rest in the initial phases.
  - If the arterial vessels become completely occluded, the patient often experiences pain at rest, ulceration, or gangrene (wet or dry).

Risk Factors for PAOD

- Age: for individuals older than 50 years, the risk factors for PAOD are not clear and most likely are not a direct cause of PAOD
- Tobacco use
  — Most predictive risk factor
  — 80% to 90% of individuals with symptomatic PAOD report using tobacco
  — Nicotine and cotinine (primary nicotine metabolite) adversely affect the vasculature
    - Primary endothelial injury
      ○ Sloughing of endothelial cells
      ○ Hyperplastic response leads to thickening of arterial wall

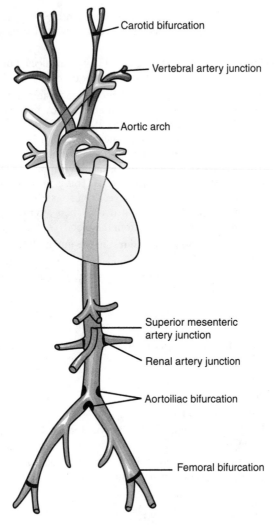

Figure 5–3 Common sites of occlusions in arteriosclerosis obliterans.

- Growth of arthromatous lesions
  - Increased levels of circulating lipids and free fatty acids
  - Increased concentrations of the "arthrogenic" lipoproteins—low-density lipoproteins (LDL) and very-low-density lipoproteins (VLDL)
  - Increased production of growth factors and collagen leads to plaque enlargement
  - Increased levels of carbon monoxide lead to increased endothelial permeability
  - Altered production of factors affecting platelet adhesion lead to increased platelet aggregation
- Increased smooth muscle tone (vasoconstriction)
  - Increased production of vasoconstrictive agents (thromboxane A_2)
  - Decreased production of vasodilator agent (prostacyclin or PG_{12})
- Increased blood viscosity
  - Elevated hematocrit, white blood cells (WBC), and fibrinogen levels leads to increased blood viscosity and decreased rate of blood flow.[1]
- Raises blood lipids and negatively affects the peripheral flow)

- Diabetes mellitus: 7% to 30% of patients with diabetes have occlusive disease; PAOD is more extensive in younger (age 50 years and under) patients with diabetes; there is a tendency for less involvement of the aorta and iliac arteries and more involvement of the popliteal and tibial arteries. The longer the patient has diabetes, the more likely arterial occlusion will occur.

  — Important prognostic variables include:
    - Increased plaque formation
    - Increased RBC rigidity
    - Increased blood viscosity and coagulability
    - Hypertrophy of vascular smooth muscle
    - Increased vascular resistance

— These patients commonly have multisegmental occlusions

— These patients commonly have multivessel disease

— PAOD is usually bilateral versus unilateral in nondiabetics

— PAOD patients with diabetes are poor candidates for angioplasty due to their small size of vessels most often involved

- Hyperinsulinemia and insulin resistance

   — May contribute to hypertrophy of vascular smooth muscle and increased vascular resistance—insulin is a vascular growth factor

   — Elevated insulin levels may explain PAOD development in nondiabetics

- Hyperlipoproteinemia: occurs in 31% to 57% of patients, the exact causal relationship is unknown

- Homocystinuria is a rare autosomal dominant disease with early onset severe atherosclerosis that:

   — Contributes to endothelial injury and platelet aggregation

   — Can be normalized with vitamin B_6, B_{12}, and folic acid administration

- Hypertension: systolic hypertension is prevalent; occurs in 29% to 39% of patients due to the constant, excessive, turbulent pressure that causes intimal arterial damage

   — Hypertension is the second most predictive risk factor for PAOD and causes:[1]

     ▪ Increased production of vascular smooth muscle

     ▪ Activation of the renin-angiotension-aldosterone system

     ▪ Increased arteriolar sodium transport

     ▪ High intracellular production of factors contributing to vasoconstriction

     ▪ Increased interaction between the endothelium and the circulating blood elements

   — 60% to 70% of individuals with occlusive disease have two of the last six risk factors listed above.

- Buerger's disease (thromboangiitis obliterans) is the second most common cause of chronic arterial occlusion.

  — It occurs in young adults who are heavy smokers— exclusively limited to this population—especially males.

  — It causes an intense inflammatory process—possibly autoimmune—leading to occlusion of the arteries and veins. The midsized arteries and veins are affected first and the progression of the disease is proximal.

  — Cold sensitivity, ulcers, and gangrene occur in the upper and lower extremities.

  — Marginal collateral circulation of toes and fingers causes early tissue necrosis with occlusion.

  — Ulceration may occur spontaneously but more commonly follows minor trauma.

  — Symptoms are always bilateral, frequently involving all four limbs.

  — Necrotizing vasculitides are the less common causes of ischemic wounds. They are a broad group of disorders with:

    ▪ Inflammatory reactions in the blood vessels causing necrosis and destruction of the vessel wall such as Takayasu's arteritis, polyarteritis nodosa, rheumatoid arthritis, and system lupus erythematosus.

- Sickle cell anemia is another cause of occlusion, affecting both the arterial and venous systems at a microvascular level.

  — The majority of ulcerations are closely associated with venous insufficiency but arterial ulcers may also occur.

Nursing Assessment

- If the patient has a lower extremity ulcer, it is necessary to assess for arterial disease.[2]
- Arterial ulcer clinical characteristics include:[5,3]

  — Skin color

  — Elevational pallor: more advanced lesions require less elevation to obtain the same results; elevation causes ischemia from the maximal cutaneous dilatation and when the limb is returned to the dependent position, returning blood flow causes an intense red, reactive hyperemia.

— Dependent rubor: cyanotic, purple discoloration of the extremity with dependency; occurs due to reduced inflow; therefore, blood in the capillaries is stagnant and oxygen extraction high; hemoglobin becomes deoxygenated causing capillary blood to appear blue.

— Occurs in any part of leg but more common below the ankle, on tips of the digits, or between digits

— Reduced or absent pulses: dorsalis pedis and/or post tibial; arteries often feel hard and rubbery; collateral circulation rarely produces a palpable pulse distal to an occlusion

---

 Nursing Tip
Decreased or absent palpable pedal pulses necessitates a referral to a vascular physician for further evaluation.[2] If Trancutanteous oxygen tension (TcPO2) is below 40 mmHg the patient should also be referred for further evaluation as this may be an indicator of impaired healing.[2]

— Skin temperature of the extremity is usually decreased; this is most critically important when there is a profound difference between the more and less ischemic limbs

— Ulcers are usually small in size and commonly occur on a toe or at a traumatic injury site; the ulcers are small craters with well defined borders with a 'punched out' (punctuate) appearance

— Edema is localized, if present

— Hemosiderin (brown) staining is NEVER present unless mixed disease occurs

— Necrotic tissue is common: gangrene wet and/or dry; necrosis of the limb will continue past the ulcer and stops where blood supply is sufficient to maintain tissue viability

— Edges of the wound are most often sharp and well-defined; the base of the wound is usually devoid of healthy granulation tissue and the periwound skin is most often pale and mottled

  ▪ Eschar is often thickened and raised above the skin level

— Pain: present with exercise in a muscle group (calf muscles most commonly), at night (nocturnal pain), and during rest (rest pain); the patient may complain of cramping, burning, aching; pain may be relieved with dependent limb positioning and aggravated by elevation.

  ▪ Intermittent claudication: differential diagnosis is that some exertion causes the pain; however, it can mimic the pain of osteoarthritis of the hip or knee and neurospinal compression due to narrowing of the lumbar neurospinal canal from osteophytosis (spinal stenosisz)

— Nocturnal pain is caused by worsening occlusion with leg elevation and reduced cardiac output while asleep.

— Rest pain occurs in the absence of activity, with legs dependent; rest pain signals advanced disease.

— If pain is felt at rest it is usually caused by advanced arterial ischemia often resulting in gangrene and amputation. The pain at rest does not occur in a muscle group and is often described as severe burning.

— Pain usually occurs one joint distal to the occlusion (Table 5-1):

— Intermittent limping with exercise is a sign of claudication

— Some individuals perceive claudication as a "leg giving out" or "leg fatigue" rather than pain

• Skin is shiny, smooth, thin, dry, and without hair

• Toenails are thickened, may/not be mycotic

• Skin color changes with leg elevation and dependence

Table 5–1 Relation of Pain to Site of Occlusion

Site of Occlusion	Location of Pain
Ileofemoral arteries	Thighs, buttocks, calves
Superficial femoral artery	Calf
Infrapopliteal	Foot

- Supine patient, leg raised to a 60° angle for 15 to 60 seconds
  - Observe for visible color change
  - Pallor in fair-skinned individuals
  - Gray in darker-skinned individuals
  - 25 seconds equals severe occlusive disease
  - 30 seconds equals moderately severe occlusive disease
  - 45 to 60 seconds equals mild occlusive disease
- Place the leg in dependent position
  - Observe for rubor (purple-red color of the lower limb)
- Increased venous filling time
  - Elevate and then lower the limb and record the amount of time in seconds required for venous filling
    - More than 20 seconds equals severe occlusive disease
    - Prolonged venous filling time is independently predictive of PAOD
  - Muscle atrophy occurs with chronic tissue malnourishment; loss of strength in the ischemic zone is common; decreased joint mobility is also seen especially in the foot; these changes often increase the likelihood of the development of more ulcers
- Carotid or cardiac bruit: turbulent blood flow caused by vessel wall vibration; heard the loudest in systole and with greater/increased stenosis it may be heard in diastole
- Palpation of pulses
  - Compare contralaterally and proximal to distal

— Diminished or absent pulses are independently predictive of PAOD

  ▪ MUST evaluate both dorsalis pedis and posterior tibialis pulses before documenting significantly diminished or absent pulses

  ▪ Absence of both a normal dorsalis pedis and a normal posterior tibialis pulse are evidence of PAOD BUT presence of a normal pulse in either location is considered indicative of normal pedal pulses

• Capillary refill

— Press the toe pad firmly between the index finger and thumb to empty surface vessels; monitor the refill time

— Normal is less than 3 seconds

— Patients with PAOD may have normal capillary refill due to emptied vessels filling in a retrograde manner

• Skin temperature

— Compare extremities contralaterally

— Palpate lightly with palmar surface of fingers and hands from proximal to distal, right leg to left leg, right foot to left foot

— Significant findings

  ▪ Unilateral coolness indicates positive predictive value

  ▪ Sudden marked change from proximal to distal

— Wounds may be partial or full thickness

  ▪ Common locations are the distal aspects of extremities (tips of toes and fingers)

  ▪ Another common location is at pressure points of the foot (heel or lateral foot)

  ▪ Located in areas of trauma

  ▪ Wound bed is pale or necrotic and usually dry

  ▪ Minimal wound exudate

  ▪ Periwound skin: faint halo or erythema or slight fluctuance suggests infection

DIAGNOSTIC PROCEDURES

Noninvasive Testing

- Segmental extremity pressure measurement
  - Quick screening test: resting systolic blood pressure taken at the brachial artery and the posterior artery or the dorsal foot artery. Ankle brachial index (ABI) or ankle arm index (AAI) is then calculated through dividing the pressure obtained at the ankle by the pressure obtained at the brachial arterial
  - Values: differ slightly with each vascular laboratory
  - Segmental pressures can be obtained at various levels on the leg for localization of occlusive disease
    - Supine position with blood pressure cuff to high thigh, low thigh, upper calf, and ankle; commonly the bilateral brachial and ankle pressures are taken
    - Gradients of more than 20 mmHg between sites are diagnostic for occlusive disease in the intervening segment
- Toe pressure: usually a plethysmograph or laser Doppler is used
  - In diabetics, inaccurately high ABIs—due to blood vessel calcification—have been found and toe measurements are therefore more useful.
  - Normal gradient between the ankle and toe is 20 mmHg to 30 mmHg
  - Healing of distal wounds is expected when toe pressures are greater than 40 mmHg but rarely will healing occur if pressures are less than 20 mmHg; 20 mmHg to 40 mmHg is a gray zone for healing
- Doppler wave form provides an analog signal proportional to the velocity of the blood in the vessel being studied. It is the overall shape of the wave form that is diagnostic.

Treatment Issues and Challenges

- Ankle/brachial index (ABI) also known as ankle/arm index (AAI): 0.8 to 0.9 equals mild obstruction; 0.5 to 0.7 equals moderate obstruction; 0.5 equals severe obstruction

Wound care: avoid occlusive and adhesive, semiocclusive dressings; this is a conservative approach. Before topical treatment is selected evaluate:

- Perfusion status
- Goal of topical treatment
- Potential for infection
- Wound parameters (depth and exudate volume)
- Caregiver knowledge and ability

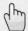

Nursing Alert

Remember: most common sensitivity reactions are to neomycin, lanolin, and parabens
- *Evaluate and treat skin maceration from exudate*
  — *Use nonalcohol skin barrier to prevent and treat (3M No Sting®)*
- *Use moisturizer twice daily and with each dressing change distal to the wound in the presence of dry skin*

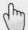

Nursing Alert

NO debridement if pulse is absent or extremity is cold

- Dry, intact, noninfected eschar serves as a bacterial barrier
  — Maintain the closed wound when:
    - Limb is clearly ischemic with limited or no potential for healing
    - No indications of infection
    - Wound surface is dry and necrotic
    - Frequently monitor for any signs and symptoms of deterioration of wound status (infection signs and symptoms)

— Paint with antiseptic solution such as povidone iodine 10% and allow to dry
— Apply dry gauze dressing
— NO tape or adhesives to skin

- Treat if signs and symptoms of infection or cellulitus occur:
  — Increased pain
  — Increased necrosis
  — Fluctuance of periwound skin
  — Erythematous halo (faint) around wound or necrotic area
  — Treatment
    ▪ Antibiotics (systemic may be necessary) and culture-based
    ▪ Aggressive and early debridement of necrotic tissue requires an immediate referral to a surgeon, podiatrist, nurse practitioner, or physician assistant for sterile surgical debridement
      ○ NOT with semipermeable or occlusive dressings
    ▪ Elimination of dead space in the wound through wound packing; use loose NOT tight packing
    ▪ Meticulous wound care is necessary
  — When wounds are infected, dressings require changing once a day minimally and before strike through has occurred

Nursing Alert
Compression is usually contraindicated

- Revascularization is the treatment of choice if the patient is an appropriate candidate; usually an AAI/ABI less than 0.5 means the wound is unlikely to heal without surgical intervention

- Patient education and considerations:
  - Eliminate constrictive clothing and constrictive positions
    - Wear socks during cold weather to prevent vasoconstriction
  - Avoid cool temperatures
  - Avoid heating devices, hot water bottles, heating pads, or other thermal devices
    - Always check water temperature with hand or elbow before bathing
  - Avoid injuries and trauma to all extremities
    - Avoid walking barefoot even indoors
    - Wear consistent protective foot gear (closed-toe, closed-heel)
    - Inspect foot gear routinely before wearing
    - Careful fitting of foot gear to prevent pressure, friction, and shear
    - Use protective shin guards when working around home or yard
    - NO "bathroom" surgery; seek professional treatment; limit self-care of nails to conservative trimming and filing
    - Do NOT use antiseptic or chemical corn and callous removers
    - Inspect feet and legs twice daily for injury and trauma; seek timely professional help if such injury or trauma is noted
  - Regulate blood sugars
  - Evaluate the patient holistically including nutrition and hydration status
  - Exercise to tolerance; encourage mobility and ambulation using a planned, graduated walking program
    - Physiologic benefits
      - Adaptive changes in ischemic tissues resulting in improved oxygen use at cellular level

- Enhanced workload tolerance
- Decreased blood viscosity
- Decreased blood pressure
- Weight loss
- Stress reduction
- Improved gait efficiency
- Reduced pain
- Improved exercise tolerance

- Maintain legs in a neutral position; do not elevate above heart level
  - Avoid crossing legs
- Use bed and foot cradle taking care with the insensate limb
- Skin care twice daily
  - Use gentle, pH-balanced cleanser
  - Moisturizer/emollient after bathing to prevent cracking and fissures
  - Dry carefully between toes whenever moisture collects after bathing and swimming
  - Use lamb's wool or foam toe "sleeves" to prevent interdigital friction and pressure
- Pressure reduction and relief must be accomplished
- Quit tobacco use
- If the patient has a graft, educate him or her to:
  - Monitor the graft site by palpating pulses and reporting significant changes promptly on a daily basis
  - Recognize reportable signs and symptoms of graft failure
  - Continue behaviors that promote vascular health

Box 5-1 Arterial Wound Care

Intact, dry necrotic tissue such as eschar and dry gangrene

- Keep dry and intact as long as possible
- Paint with antiseptic solution (povidone iodine 10% solution)
  — Allow to air dry
  — Cover with nonshearing dressing
  — Do not apply adhesives to skin
  — Change dressing daily and evaluate the limb
- Pressure reduction and relief

Wet, moist necrotic tissue

- Debridement (surgical is the best option)
- Meticulous wound care to avoid infection post debridement
- No occlusive, semiocclusive, or adhesive dressings
- Cleanse gently with normal saline or wound cleanser
  — Protect periwound skin from excessive moisture
  — May use nonalcohol skin barrier wipe up to wound edge to decrease maceration
- Hydrogel (sparingly) to wound bed to maintain moist wound healing
- Cover with dry dressing (nonstick gauze is best)
- Moisturize dry skin distal to the wound

Dry wound bed

- Meticulous wound care to avoid infection
- Do not use occlusive, semiocclusive, or adhesive dressings

- Cleanse gently with normal saline or wound cleanser

  — Protect periwound skin from excessive moisture

  — May use nonalcohol skin barrier wipe up to wound edge to decrease maceration

- Hydrogel (sparingly) to wound bed to maintain moist wound healing

  — Cover with dry dressing (nonstick gauze is best)

  — Moisturize dry skin distal to the wound

  — Change dressing as clinical symptoms indicate

Infected wound

- Notify physician immediately

  — Goal is to improve circulation without amputation if possible

- Wound culture and biopsy

- Systemic or topical antibiotics based on organisms present

- Meticulous wound care to avoid spreading infection

- Do not use occlusive, semiocclusive, or adhesive dressings

- Cleanse gently with normal saline or wound cleanser (avoid use of more caustic cleansers)

  — Protect periwound skin from excessive moisture

  — May use nonalcohol skin barrier wipe up to wound edge to eliminate maceration

- Use hydrogel or topical antibiotic(sparingly) to wound bed to maintain moist wound healing

  — Bactroban

  — Iodosorb gel

- Cover with dry dressing (nonstick gauze is best)

- Moisturize dry skin distal to the wound

- Change every day at a minimum

- Educate patients and caregivers regarding signs and symptoms to report

Note: Discuss addition of dietary supplemental arginine with the physician and dietician. Small studies have indicated that arginine-supplemented diet can increase the level of polyamines and therefore promote tissue repair.

REFERENCES

1. Bryant RA. *Acute and Chronic Wounds.* 2nd ed. St. Louis, MO: Mosby; 2000.
2. Hopf HW, et al. Guidelines for the treatment of arterial insufficiency ulcers. *Wound Repair and Regeneration.* 2006;14;693–710.
3. Nick J, London M, Donnelly R. ABCs of arterial and venous disease: Ulcerated lower limb. *BMJ.* 2000;320:1589–1591.
4. Rowe V. Peripheral arterial occlusive disease. Available at: http:www.emedicine.com/MED/topic391.htm. Accessed January 5, 2008.
5. Verhaeghe R. Epidemiology and prognosis of peripheral obliterative arteriopathy. *Drugs.* 1998;56(suppl 3):S1.

SUGGESTED READING

Baranoski S, Ayello E. *Wound Care Essentials Practice Principles.* Philadelphia, PA: Lippincott Williams & Wilkins 2004.
Goldstein D, Mureebe L, Kerstein, M. Differential diagnosis: assessment of the lower-extremity ulcer—is it arterial, venous, neuropathic? *Wounds.* 1998;10(4):125–131.
Hess CT. *Wound Care.* 2nd ed. Springhouse, PA:Springhouse Corp; 1998.
Hess CT. *Wound Care.* 3rd ed. Springhouse, PA: Springhouse Corp;. 2000.

Hilleman D. Management of peripheral arterial disease. *American Journal of Health Syst Pharm*. 1998;55(suppl 1):S21.

Lopez AP, et al. Venous ulcers. *Wounds*. 1998;10(5):149.

Mahler GD, et al, eds.*Clinician's Pocket Guide to Chronic Wound Repair*. Springhouse, PA: Springhouse Corp; 1999.

Scanlon VC, et al. *Essentials of Anatomy and Physiology*. 3rd ed. Philadelphia, PA: FA Davis; 1999.

Seaman S. Evaluation and management of lower extremity ulcers: adherence to prescribed therapy can save limbs. *Advance for Nurse Practitioners*. Mar 2002;10(3):32–47.

Seidel H, Ball J, Dains J, Benedict GW.. *Mosby's Guide to Physical Examination*. 4th ed.. St Louis, MO: Mosby; 1999.

Stalano-Coico, et al. Wound Fluids: A reflection of the state of healing. *Ostomy/Wound Management*. January 2000;46 (suppl 1A)S85–93.

Sussman C, Bates-Jensen B. *Wound Care A Collaborative Practice Manual for Physical Therapists and Nurses*. Gaithersburg, MD: Aspen Publications; 1998.

Support Systems International, Inc. *The Skin*, Module 1. Charleston, SC: Hillenbrand; 1993.

Swartz M. *Textbook of Physical Diagnosis History and Examination*. 3rd ed. Philadelphia, PA: W.B. Saunders; 1998.

Terry M, et al. Tobacco: its impact on vascular disease. *Surg Clin North Amer*. 1998;78(3)409.

Tierney L, McPhee S, Papadakis M. *Current Medical Diagnosis and Treatment*. 37th ed. Stamford, CT: Appleton & Lange; 1998.

WOCN Guidance on OASIS Skin and Wound Status MO Items. Available at: http://www. deroyal.com/Wound_Care. Accessed May 24, 2001.

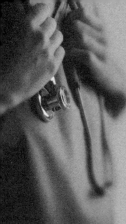

Chapter 6

NEUROPATHIC AND DIABETIC ULCER ASSESSMENT AND MANAGEMENT PRINCIPLES

KEY POINTS

- Peripheral neuropathy is a risk factor for developing ulcers and complicates healing.
- Diabetes is included within neuropathic disorders, however not the only cause.
- Management of the patient with neuropathic ulcers includes complete pressure relief, management of infection, topical treatment, and prevention of trauma.
- Patient education for long- and short-term management and prevention of new wounds or reoccurrence should be part of the plan of care.

PERIPHERAL NEUROPATHY: ETIOLOGY

Peripheral neuropathy is a common disorder that occurs as a result of damage to the peripheral nerves. It can result from local trauma such as bone fractures and compartment syndrome, or in relation to systemic diseases.

The medical conditions that may contribute to peripheral neuropathy include:

- Diabetes
- Mechanical pressure (compression or entrapment)
- Direct trauma
- Penetrating injuries
- Contusions
- Fractures or dislocated bones
- Pressure on superficial nerves (ulnar, radial, or peroneal)
- Interneural hemorrhage
- Cold exposure
- Radiation
- Vascular or collagen disorders (atherosclerosis, systemic lupus erythematosis, scleroderma, sarcoidosis, rheumatoid arthritis, polyarterities nodosa, Hansen disease)

Individuals with peripheral neuropathy do not usually present with wounds as a result of the neuropathy, but rather from the pressure, trauma, or skin dryness that was not detected earlier by the patient because of the nerve damage. Therefore, it is incumbent upon the health-care provider to educate these individuals on injury prevention.

If wounds develop, it is important to determine the cause, correct the cause when possible, and treat the wounds. The evaluation process should include determining intrinsic and extrinsic wound healing factors to help formulate the plan of care. For instance, correction may include surgery or other invasive procedures, off-loading products, and systemic antibiotic therapy.

The chain of events that cause traumatic injuries to result in disability are:

- Trauma
- Inflammation
- Ulceration
- Infection
- Absorption
- Deformity
- Disability

DIABETES MELLITUS

The American Diabetic Association (ADA) defines diabetes mellitus as "a disease in which the body doesn't produce or properly use insulin."[1]

The following statistics demonstrate the extent of diabetes in the United States:

- 7% of the American population has diabetes, or an estimated 20.8 million Americans[1]
- Only 14.6 million Americans have been diagnosed with diabetes[1]
- 6.2 million Americans are unaware they have diabetes[1]
- 54 million Americans have prediabetes[1]

- 5% to 10% of diabetics have Type 1 diabetes[1]
  — Type 1 diabetes is an autoimmune disorder that causes destruction of pancreatic ß-cells and requires insulin therapy to prevent complications[1]
  — Type 1 diabetes has an abrupt onset of symptoms including hyperglycemia and ketoacidosis[1]
  — The pathophysiologic insult of type 1 diabetes is slow and progressive
- Most Americans have type 2 diabetes
- 90% to 95% of diabetics have type 2 diabetes[1]
  — Type 2 diabetes is a relative insulin deficiency due to the failure to make enough insulin or the inability to utilize existing insulin properly
  — Approximately 30% of type 2 diabetics are undiagnosed[1]
  — Severe insulin resistance may exist for years before diagnosis and treatment of type 2 diabetes is made
  — Type 2 diabetes is highest among:
    - African Americans
    - Hispanics
    - Native Americans
    - Asian Americans
  — **The incidence of type 2 diabetes has increased 48% in the last decade**[1,2]
    - 70% of these individuals are aged 30 years or younger[2]
- Type 2 diabetes is the single **most common cause of lower extremity amputations**[1]
- Foot problems are one of most common complications that result in the hospitalization of diabetics, equaling 20% to 25% of all hospital stays for diabetics[2]
- Approximately 120,000 nontraumatic amputations of the lower extremities are performed every year[3]
  — 45% to 83% of these amputations are performed on diabetics[3,4]

- The risk of lower extremity amputation is 15 to 46 times greater in diabetics than in nondiabetics
- The risk of reamputation after initial amputation or amputation of the contralateral extremity is high in diabetics
  — 9% to 17% of diabetic patients experiencing a lower extremity amputation will have a second amputation in the same year[2]
  — 25% to 68% of diabetics will have a contralateral amputation within 3 to 5 years of the first amputation[3–5]
- The 5-year survival rate postamputation is 41% to 70%[3,4,6,7]
- 75% to 83% of all amputations among African Americans, Hispanics, and Native Americans have diabetes as a contributing factor[3,5–7]
  — The incidence of lower extremity amputations compared to non-Hispanic whites is:
    - 1.5 times higher in Hispanics[3,5,6,8,9]
    - 2.1 times higher in African Americans[3,5,6,8,9]
- The arterial and venous systems are essentially the same anatomically in diabetics and nondiabetics

Arterial Occlusion in Diabetes

Of those individuals with diabetes mellitus, 7% to 30% have occlusive disease at a younger age and have more extensive disease than those without diabetes mellitus. There is a tendency for less involvement of the aorta and iliac arteries and more involvement of the popliteal and tibial arteries in this population. The longer the individual has the disease the more likely arterial occlusion will occur.[10–13]

- Important prognostic variables for arterial occlusion in the presence of diabetes mellitus include:
  — Increased plaque formation
  — Increased red blood cell (RBC) rigidity
  — Increased blood viscosity and coagulability

— Hypertrophy of vascular smooth muscle

— Increased vascular resistance

* Multisegmental occlusions are common
* Multivessel disease is common
* Arterial disease is usually bilateral versus unilateral in nondiabetics
* Diabetics are poor candidates for angioplasty because of their small vessel size
* The underlying pathology is usually not reversible; therefore, the disease processes affecting the diabetic wound will generally worsen over time

NEUROPATHIC/DIABETIC ULCERS

Assessment of neurologic and musculoskeletal conditions should include measurement of sensory, autonomic, and motor neuropathy and the shape of the feet for callous, edema, and deformities. An assessment of the client's foot gear should also be performed to assess for areas of tightness or calluses on the client's feet. In addition the foot gear should be assessed for unusual wear patterns on the sole and heel areas.

Clients should be asked for an approximate date of their last foot gear fitting, what size foot gear they have worn in the past, the size foot gear they are currently wearing, and when was the last time they purchased new foot gear.

Nursing Assessment

Nursing Alert
The highest recurrence of ulcerations occur over previous sites of ulceration.

* Patient History: Include history of sensation changes in the hands and feet including any present symptoms.

- Risk factors for neuropathic/diabetic ulcers include:
  — Peripheral sensory neuropathy
  — Structural foot deformity
  — Trauma and improperly fitting shoes
  — Callus formation
  — History of prior ulcers
  — Prolonged, elevated pressures
  — Limited joint mobility
  — Uncontrolled hyperglycemia
  — Duration of diabetes
  — Blindness or partial eyesight
  — Chronic renal disease
  — Older age (65 years and older)
- Risk factors for amputation are:
  — Peripheral sensory neuropathy
  — Vascular insufficiency
  — Infection
  — History of foot ulcer or amputation
  — Structural foot deformity
  — Trauma
  — Charcot deformity
  — Impaired vision
  — Poor glycemic control
  — Poor footwear
  — Older age (65 years and older)
  — Male gender
  — Ethnicity
- There are two major groups of peripheral neuropathy:

  1. Gradual onset of peripheral neuropathy
     - Usually painless
     - Unknown cause, but may be due to duration of diabetes and above normal blood glucose levels

- Symptoms include:
  - Numbness
  - Tingling
  - Burning
  - Pins and needles sensation

2. Sudden onset and disappearance of peripheral neuropathy
   - Develops suddenly; may be due to hyperglycemia
   - Symptoms include:
     - Always painful
     - When pain disappears, it leaves sensory loss

- In the diabetic, limb ulceration and tissue destruction is brought about by four types of stress:

1. Ischemic necrosis
   - Usually on the lateral aspect of the 5th metatarsal head
   - Often caused by a shoe that is too narrow
   - Caused by continuous low pressure to an area over long time periods resulting in tissue death

2. Mechanical disruption
   - High pressure (600 psi) causes direct injury with immediate tissue damage
   - May be caused by chemical skin damage
   - Injury caused by stepping on a foreign object

1. Inflammatory destruction
   - Repetitive pressures (40–60 psi) cause inflammation that weakens the tissue
   - Leads to callus formation and finally ulceration from the repetition (walking on the same area repetitively)

2. Osteomyelitis or other infections
   - Tissue destruction is caused by moderate force in the affected limb in the presence of infection
   - Infection is spread as the forces are applied by intermittent pressure

> **Nursing Tip**
> *Instruct the caregiver or the patient to perform foot and skin inspections daily whether the patient has an ulcer or not. This is a very important preventative intervention as the patient with a neuropathic ulcer may not feel pain and will continue to walk or otherwise place pressure on the injured area that continues to cause damage to the tissue. Alternatively, the person with normal sensation will feel pain and will subsequently avoid placing continued pressure and stress on the injured area. Assess the patient and caregivers for understanding of this concept.*

Physical Assessment

The clinical characteristics of neuropathic/diabetic ulcers must be assessed including:

- Location: may occur on any part of the leg; most commonly seen on the plantar aspect of the foot, metatarsal heads, heels, trauma sites, and areas of altered pressure points
- Size: often very small in size with even, well-defined edges
- Edema: localized if present and generally early in the ulcer progression
- Pain: usually painless
- Common orthopedic changes: plantar flexion contractures, hammertoes, or Charcot foot—a progressive condition that affects bones and all tissues of the lower extremity that occurs after denervation of a joint and results in the structural change of the foot causing a convex midfoot arch; the actual cause is controversial
- Skin color changes: never hemosiderin staining (brown staining of the leg) unless mixed disease—venous and arterial
- Skin characteristics: surrounding skin is often dry with fissures and callus formation

Table 6-1 Wagner Scale for Grading Neuropathic Ulcers

Grade	Description
Grade 0	Skin intact
Grade 1	Superficial ulcer
Grade 2	Deeper ulcer to tendon or bone
Grade 3	Ulcer has abscess or osteomyelitis
Grade 4	Gangrene on forefoot
Grade 5	Gangrene over major portion of foot

Reproduced with permission from Wagner FEW: The dysvascular foot: a system for diagnosis and treatment. *Foot and Ankle.* 2:64–122. Copyright © 2008 by the American Orthopaedic Foot and Ankle Society, Inc.

- The Wagner scale helps the clinician effectively grade neuropathic ulcers (Table 6-1).

  Other physical assessment techniques include:
- Check vital signs and report hypertension
  — Report any findings that fall outside of baseline
- Check pedal and post tibial pulses
- Check foot and limb warmth
- Check blood sugar levels since last visit
- Assess patient and caregiver education regarding daily foot care and response
- Perform wound care with very clean technique
- Be sure to thoroughly document all of this information in the patient record

Treatment and Management

The nurse relies on collaboration with the multidisciplinary team to assist in the treatment and management of neuropathic/diabetic ulcers. It is important that the nurse clearly documents each treatment and related evaluation to help the health-care team formulate and execute an effective plan of care (POC).

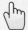

Nursing Alert
It is of extreme importance to treat immediately any minor injuries or trauma in the neuropathic (and often diabetic) foot to prevent further tissue damage. Lack of recognition of the injury or injury type and inappropriate treatment or delay in treatment can lead to amputation.

The primary treatment goals in managing neuropathic/diabetic ulcers are to prevent limb loss and maintain quality of life.

The nurse works to prevent limb loss and to maintain the patient's quality of life through:

• Appropriate screening and examination
• Prevention measures to avoid ulceration and recurrence
• Early recognition and treatment of diabetic/neuropathic foot complications
• Patient and caregiver education of the above
• Table 6–2 summarizes the evaluation, assessment, and management of diabetic ulcers
• The nurse obtains explicit orders for off-loading from the physician including:
  — Total nonweightbearing, crutches, bedrest, or wheelchair
  — Total contact casting
  — Foot casts or boots
  — Removable walking braces with rocker bottom soles
  — Total contact orthoses; custom walking braces
  — Patellar tendon-bearing braces
  — Half shoes or wedge shoes
  — Healing sandal; surgical shoe with molded plastizote insole or insert
  — Accommodative dressings: felt, foam, or felted foam
  — Shoe cutouts (toe box, medial, lateral, or dorsal pressure points)

Table 6–2   Evaluation, Assessment, and Management of
Neuropathic/Diabetic Ulcers

Evaluation/Assessment	Management
Identify major etiological factor(s)	Eliminate/control etiological factors
Identify any other factors inhibiting healing (e.g., inadequate blood sugar control)	Eliminate/control inhibitory factors
Thoroughly assess all wound characteristics	Select appropriate treatment routine (includes dressings)
Develop a POC that is individualized to the patient/caregiver/family	Monitor progress (photographs when possible)
	Educate patient/caregiver regarding maintenance of healed skin

— Assistive devices: crutches, walker, or cane

— At any time during the process, the nurse considers refer-
ring the patient to physical therapy as indicated.

• Off-loading devices help decrease pressure, neuropathy, and
ischemia. Table 6–3 demonstrates the differences among
pressure, neuropathy, and ischemia.

Topical Wound Management

The primary goal of topical wound management is to change a
chronic wound into an acute wound.

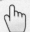

Nursing Tip
*Proceed with caution if an ulcer on a neuropathic limb
has dry eschar without signs or symptoms of infection.
The goal for this wound is to protect the eschar by
keeping it dry and free from pressure. By removing the
eschar, the wound status could change from dry and
stable to open and chronic, thus making treatment
more labor- and time-intensive.*

Table 6–3   Differences Among Pressure, Neuropathy, and Ischemia

Pressure and Neuropathy Symptoms	Ischemia Symptoms
Warm, dry, cracked skin (often pink in lightly pigmented areas)	Dry, cool skin
Callous	Absent hair
Pulses present	Reduced/absent pulses
Foot deformities (hammertoes, etc)	Inadequate capillary filling
Limited joint mobility	Positive Buerger test
Reduced/absent ankle reflexes	
Reduced/absent sensation	
Reduced/absent vibration sense	

- The most common treatment applications for neuropathic/diabetic ulcers are:
  — Hydrogel: applicable when wound is dry to minimally draining only; use care not to macerate (wet) the peri-wound skin.
  — Foam: applicable when wound has moderate to large exudate amounts and the wound bed is clean. Do not use on dry wounds.
  — Hydrocolloids: use when wound has low to moderate exudate. Do not use with heavy exudate, sinus tracts, or wounds requiring debridement or packing. Do not use over infected wounds.
  — Alginates: applicable for heavily exudative wounds. Do not use with minimal to moderate exudate.
  — Collagen dressings: applicable for low to heavily draining wounds. These dressings have an animal source and may not be acceptable to patients who are vegetarian, or who have personal, religious, or allergic prohibitions against the use of animal products.

— Antimicrobial dressings: applicable for infected or clean wounds to prevent infection (usually silver- or iodine-based). Do not use on patients who have allergies to components.

— Detergents/antiseptics (povidone iodine): applicable for contaminated or infected wounds. Not intended for use with healthy, granulating wounds.

— Topical antibiotics (silver sulfadiazine, Bacitracin, Bactroban [MRSA]): used in contaminated or infected wounds, not with healthy, granulating wounds.

— Enzymes: use with care and in short duration with frequent evaluation of wound condition.

— Growth factors (Beclaplermin gel {Regranex}, autologous platelets): used in neuropathic diabetic foot ulcers, not with infected wounds or necrotic wounds.

— Dermal/skin substitutes: used in venous stasis ulcers and diabetic foot ulcers, not with infected or necrotic wounds.

Treatment Principles of Neuropathic/Diabetic Ulcers

The following treatment principles are effective in treating and managing neuropathic/diabetic ulcers.

• Stabilize blood sugars

— Hyperglycemia affects immunologic defenses, granulocyte adherence, chemotaxis, phagocytosis, and bactericidal function

— Some type 2 diabetics must go on insulin during the treatment of the ulceration(s) to achieve healing to control blood glucose levels

• Control infection

— Diabetic feet tend to be polymicrobial; however, cellulitus of nonulcerated skin is usually caused by *Staphylococcus aureus* (occasionally a gram negative bacilli will cause this also)

— Common pathogens that contribute to infection are:

▪ Staphylococcus aureus

▪ Coagulase negative staphylococci

▪ Enterococci

- Group B streptococci
- Proteus
- Escherichia coli
- Klebsiella
- Enterobacter
- Pseudomonas aeruginosa
- Bacteroides (anaerobe)
- Clostridium (anaerobe)
- Peptococcus (anaerobe)
- Peptostreptococcus (anaerobe)
- Tinea species (fungus)
— Mild infection causes:
  - Localized cellulitus
  - Superficial ulceration
  - Minimal purulence
  - No systemic signs or symptoms
— Moderate infection causes:
  - Cellulitus of foot or ankle
  - Deep or penetrating ulceration
  - Plantar abscess
  - Acute osteomyelitis
  - Systemic signs or symptoms
— Severe infection causes:
  - Proximal cellulitis, lymphangitis
  - Gangrene, necrotizing fasciitis
  - Clinical septicemia

• Rule out osteomyelitis; present in one-third to two-thirds of diabetic patients with moderate to severe pedal infections.[14]
  — Most likely to occur with puncture wounds
  — Occurs in those patients with a history of a chronically draining wound
  — Present when exposed bone is at the base of an ulcer

— Erythrocyte sedimentation rate (ESR) of 70 to 100 mm/hr is predictive of osteomyelitis.[14]
— X-ray is not the best diagnostic tool
— Bone biopsy is usually definitive
— CT scan or Indium-111-labeled leukocyte scanning is definitive but costly
— Treatment usually requires 4 to 6 weeks of antibiotic therapy (may be longer in some cases)

> **Nursing Alert**
> *Treatment of moderate to severe infections should be evaluated immediately by a physician.*

— Treatment of infection may include:
   ▪ Systemic oral or intravenous antibiotics
   ▪ Debridement of necrotic tissue
   ▪ Incision and drainage, soft tissue/bone/joint resection
   ▪ Amputation
• Eliminate weight bearing and pressure
   — Ideal is total removal of weight on foot and complete bed rest in recalcitrant wounds
   — "Healing" sandals or special shoes
   — Total contact casts
   — Removable walking casts
• Correct ischemia
   — Hyperbaric oxygen therapy (not a substitute for revascularization)
   — Physician evaluation for revascularization
• Wound care
   — Debridement as necessary (sharp or surgical); callus removal if necessary

— Dressings that provide warm, moist environment free from external contamination (saline, hydrocolloids, alginates, foams, films, and hydrogels)

— Growth factors such as becaplermin (Regranex), a recombinant human platelet derived growth factor

— Pressure reduction

— Infection control

— Control edema if present using elevation and paste wraps. Use the following only after consultation with the physician to be sure that the patient has adequate vasculature to support use of these products: elastic support stockings and pneumatic compression pumps

• Manage gangrene

— Dry gangrene: results from loss of nourishment to the tissues; black, shriveled, and mummified tissue with a specific well-defined line of demarcation; will autoamputate in many cases

  ▪ Painting with povidone iodine and allowing this to dry often prevents progression to wet gangrene.

  ▪ Protection from destructive forces of shear and/or friction is necessary.

  ▪ Obtain a physician order for any activity that causes moistening of dry gangrene; use caution in this situation.

— Wet gangrene: caused by necrosis and destruction of tissue from excessive moisture; bacterial gases accumulate in the tissues; limb is usually painful, purple, and swollen without a well-defined line of demarcation; wet gangrene is almost always infected and requires surgical referral

— Table 6–4 demonstrates the Wagner ulcer grading scale with corresponding treatment

• Patient adherence with medical regimen including prevention strategies (Table 6–5):

Table 6–4   Wagner Ulcer Grading Scale

Grade	Treatment
0	Extra-depth shoe and insert
1	Cast or Plastizote healing shoe reduces weight to ulcer; antibiotics as required
2	Debridement and cast; antibiotics as required
3	Remove infected tissue and cast; antibiotics as required

Source: Data from Giugla M, Mulder G. The Diabetic Foot. In Medical Management of Foot Ulcers in Chronic Wound Care: A Clinical Source Book for Healthcare Professionals. Krasner D, ed. Mosby Health/Managment Publications, Inc., © 1990, pp. 223-239 and Wagner FW Jr. A classification and treatment program for diabetic, neuropathic and dysvascular foot problems. Am Acad Ortho Surg Inst Course Lect 1979;28:143–165.

- Shoes in diabetic foot care
    - Shoes should be shaped for the patient's foot type (not for fashion)
    - Shoes should have adequate length, width, and depth without compression on the toes
    - The best shoes are made of soft leather (uppers) with resilient, thick, flexible soles
    - The ball of the foot should rest in the widest part of the shoe
    - New shoes should initially be worn around the home for approximately 1 hour on a carpeted surface to evaluate for "hot" spots or other problem areas
    - Each patient should have a minimum of two pairs of shoes; wear one pair, then alternate with the other pair the next day
    - Replace shoes at regular intervals, whenever signs of wear develop
    - Feet should be measured at each shoe purchase
    - A new pair of shoes should never be worn for more than 2 hours without evaluating the feet for pressure areas
    - The maximum amount of time to wear any shoes is 5 hours.[15]

Table 6–5   Patient Prevention of Foot Ulcers

Prevention	Foot Care
Blood sugar control.	Regular podiatry visits.
Appropriate foot gear that fits properly.	Cleanse feet gently everyday.
Evaluate for ischemia, neuropathy, abnormal or changed foot structure, poor hygiene.	Gently dry feet, especially between toes.
Educate and encourage proper foot care.	Inspect feet twice a day; on arising and retiring for the day.
	Cut nails straight across. Do not cut cuticles, corns, or calluses.
	Do not use over-the-counter products or home remedies to remove calluses or corns without checking with physician, podiatrist, or nurse practitioner.
	Inspect foot gear daily and repair as necessary. DO NOT wear if not in good repair. ALWAYS wear shoes with a hard sole. Each time foot gear is to be worn, first check the inside of the shoe for any foreign objects that can cause injury.

REFERENCES

1. Available at the web site of American Diabetes Association (ADA). http://www.diabetes.org/about-diabetes.jsp. Accessed February 25, 2007.
2. World Health Organization (2002). *World Health Organization Fact Sheet No. 236: Diabetes: the Cost of Diabetes*. Retrieved December 02, 2005, from http://www.who.int/mediacentre/factsheets/fs236/en.

3. Armstrong DG, et al. Off-loading the diabetic foot wound: a randomized clinical trial. *Diabetes Care*. 2001;24: 1019–1022.

4. Broersma A. Preventing amputations in patients with diabetes and chronic kidney disease. *Nephrology Nursing Journal*; 2004:31(1):53–64.

5. Boyko EJ, Ahroni JH, Stensel V, Forsberg RC, Davignon DR, Smith DG. A prospective study of risk factors for diabetic foot ulcer. *Diabetes Care*. 1999;22(7):1036–1042.

6. Blackwell B, Aldridge R,, Jacob S. A comparison of plantar pressure in patients with diabetic foot ulcers using different hosiery. *Lower Extremity Wounds*. 2002;1(3):174–178.

7. Boulton A. Pressure and the diabetic foot: clinical science and off-loading techniques. *American Journal of Surgery*. 2004; 187:S17–S24.

8. Carrington A, et al. A foot care program for diabetic unilateral lower-limb amputees. *Diabetes Care*. 2001;24(2):216–221.

9. Cavanagh PR, Simoneau GG, Ulbrecht JS. Ulceration, unsteadiness, and uncertainty: the biomechanical consequences of diabetes mellitus. *Journal of Biomechanics*. 1993;26(suppl 1): 23–40.

10. Frykberg RA, et al. *Diabetic Foot Disorders: A Clinical Practice Guideline*. Brooklandville, MD: Data Trace Publishing Company; 2000.

11. Giurini JM. Foot complications: diagnosis and management. *International Journal of Lower Extremity Wounds*. 2005; 4(3):171–182.

12. Jeffcoate WJ, Harding KG. Diabetic foot ulcers. *The Lancet*. 2003;361:1545–1551.

13. King H, Aubert RE, Herman WH. Global burden of diabetes. *Diabetes Care*. 1998;21(9):1414–1431.

14. Kevin W, Shea MD. Antimicrobial therapy for diabetic foot infections: A practical approach. Postgraduate Medicine. July 1999;106(1). Available at, http://www.postgradmed.com/issues/1999/07_99/shea.shtml. Accessed June 6, 2007.

15. Advanced Information Series of American Diabetic Association, Inc. 1998.

SUGGESTED READING

Ahroni JH. Preventing diabetic foot complications. *Advances in Skin & Wound Care.* 2000;13:38–39. Retrieved November 1, 2005, from http://www.findarticles.com/p/artic/mi_qa3977/is_200001/ai_n889.

Aliabadi Z, Ezell OL. Preventing and treating diabetic foot ulcers. *The Clinical Advisor.* 2004; 28–32.

American Diabetes Association. Third-party reimbursement for diabetes care, self-management education, and supplies. *Diabetes Care.* 2005;28(suppl 1):S62–S63.

Caravaggi C, et al. Effectiveness and safety of a nonremovable fiberglass off-loading cast versus a therapeutic shoe in the treatment of neuropathic foot ulcers: a randomized study. *Diabetes Care.* 2000;23:1746–1751.

Cawthorne H. District assessment of diabetic foot ulceration. *Journal of Community Nursing.* 2000;5:1–6. Retrieved November 25, 2005, from http://www.jcn.co.uk?printFriend.asp?ArticleID=241.

Center for Disease Control *National Diabetes Fact Sheet*: United States 2005. Retrieved December 2, 2005, from http://www.cdc.gov.diabetes

Chakrabarty A, Norman RA, Phillips TJ. Cutaneous manifestations of diabetes. *Wounds.* 2002;14(8):267–274.

Davis M. PN plus: diabetes foot ulcers—primary care for those at risk part 4. *Practice Nurse: the Journal for Nurses in General Practice.* 2001;21(8):41 EOA.

Frykberg RG, et al. Role of neuropathy and high foot pressure in diabetic foot ulceration. *Diabetes Care.* 1998;21:714–1719.

Garrow A, Carine HM, VanSchie P, Boulton A. Efficacy of multi-layered hosiery in reducing in-shoe plantar foot pressure in high-risk patients with diabetes. *Diabetes Care.* 2005; 28:2001–2006.

Hall SJ. *Basic Biomechanics.* St. Louis, MO: Mosby Year Book; 1991.

Jude EB, Unsworth PF. Optimal treatment of infected diabetic foot ulcers. *Drugs Aging.* 2004;13:833–850.

Marks JB. The forgotten complication. *Clinical Diabetes.* 2005;23(1):3–4.

Mayfield JA, Reiber GE, Sanders LJ, Janisse D, Pogach LM. Preventive foot care in people with diabetes. *Diabetes Care.* 1998;12:2161–2177.

Ortegon MM, Redekop WK, Niessen LW. Cost-effectiveness of prevention and treatment of the diabetic foot. *Diabetes Care.* 2004;27(4):901–907.

Pham HT, Rich J, Veves A. Wound healing in diabetic foot ulcerations: a review and commentary. *Wounds.* 2000:12(4):79–81.

Praet S, Louwerens JK. The influence of shoe design on plantar pressures in neuropathic feet. *Diabetes Care.* 2003;26(2):441–445.

Russell LB. Time requirements for diabetes self-management: too much for many? *Journal of Family Practice.* 2005;1. Retrieved October 30, 2005, from http://www.findarticles.com/p/articles/mi_m0689/is_1_54/ai_n87050.

Shearer A, Adam G, Paul S, Alan O. Predicted costs and outcomes from reduced vibration detection in people with diabetes in the U.S. *Diabetes Care.* 2003:26(8):2305–2310.

Slovenkai MP. Getting—and keeping—a leg up on diabetes-related foot problems. *The Journal of Musculoskeletal Medicine.* 1998;15(12):46–55.

Stone JA. Wound healing for foot ulcers. *Diabetes Self-Management.* 2003;20(1):38–49.

Veves A, Masson EA, Fernando DJ, Boulton AJ. Use of experimental padded hosiery to reduce abnormal foot pressures in diabetic neuropathy. *Diabetes Care.* 1989:12(9):653–655.

Viswanathan V, et al. Effectiveness of different types of footwear insoles for the diabetic neuropathic foot: a follow-up study. *Diabetes Care.* 2004;27(2):474–477.

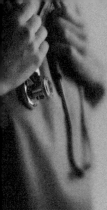

Chapter 7
LYMPHEDEMA

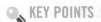

KEY POINTS

- Lymphedema is different from venous insufficiency and requires different treatment.
- There are different types of lymphedema.
- Lymphedema treatment is through management, as it cannot be cured.

ANATOMY AND PHYSIOLOGY

The lymphatic system is a one-way fluid transport system. Its capillaries receive excess interstitial fluid, proteins, cellular debris or dead cells, toxins, cancer cells, fats, and bacterial products associated with inflammation or infection. These capillaries merge into lymphatic vessels and this fluid is filtered by lymph nodes. The lymphatic system finally joins with the venous system at the thoracic duct.[1]

In the body, the net forces that drive fluid into capillaries must equal the force causing outward movement to maintain compartmental fluid balance; however, there is actually a disequilibrium that favors the outward flow of fluid.

The lymphatic capillaries are responsible for removing this extra fluid in the interstitial space. One half of total blood protein and 1 to 2 liters of water escape from the blood into the tissues every day to be returned by the lymphatic system. Lymphedema occurs when fluid (water) and proteins accumulate, and the lymphatic system is unable to mechanically remove them.

Key Definitions

Tissue fluid: fluid outside the blood and lymph vessels and capillaries.

Plasma: nonclotting fluid that makes up more than one-half of the blood; 90% water and 10% suspended particles (proteins, inorganic particles, organic substances) represents 20% of extracellular fluid volume.

Edema: abnormal or excess fluid accumulation in the interstitial space and/or tissues. This may occur anywhere in the body.

Lipedema: painless, symmetric, bilateral deposition of fat in the lower extremities almost exclusively in women (may complain of swelling in legs; however history reveals this is long standing; the swelling may change with standing and in warm environments).

Lymphedema: swelling of soft tissues, most often from poor or abnormal lymphatic system drainage.[2]

TYPES OF LYMPHEDEMA

The four main types of lymphedema are:

1. Primary lymphedema (idiopathic): most likely a congenital (born with it) disease or inherited abnormality of the lymphatic system such as a decreased number or size of lymphatic vessels (hypoplasia), or too many lymphatic vessels that do not function properly (hyperplasia). Milroy disease is a type of lymphedema that is both congenital and hereditary. It occurs more in females, and the age of onset is similar among family members.

   — Congenital: may be associated with Turner syndrome (hypoplastic lymph vessels of legs)
     - Simple: only one family member is affected
     - Milroy disease

   — Meige Disease/Lymphedema praecox (original term): spontaneously affects primarily females in the second or third decade without a known cause; onset is in the feet and often progresses upward in the body throughout life.

   — Late form (idiopathic) lymphedema forme tarde: onset occurs after age 35 with similar symptoms as praecox; females note an increase in symptoms at the time of the menses.[4]

2. Secondary lymphedema: most often the result of blocked or damaged lymphatic vessels due to surgery, radiation therapy, limb paralysis, injury, infection, and/or inflammatory disease.

— The most common cause in the United States of upper extremity lymphedema in women is surgery with radiation for breast cancer.[5]

— The most common cause in the tropical regions of the world is parasitic infections (filariasis).

3. Obstructive lymphedema:

— Malignant occlusion: occlusion or destruction of lymphatic vessels and nodes due to the malignant process or direct extension. Prostate cancer in men and lymphoma in women are the most common causes in the United States.

— Interruption of lymphatic channels or nodes due to surgery or radiation therapy: postmastectomy is the most common cause in women in the United States. It also occurs as a result of abdominal, pelvic, and external genitalia surgery such as the insertion of testicular prostheses, femoropopliteal autogenous vein bypass graft, and retroperitoneal lymphatic tuberculosis.

4. Inflammatory lymphedema:

— Due to recurrent lymphangitis or cellulitus with symptoms of:

  ▪ Sudden severe chill (may be preceded by distress to the extremity or the proximal lymph nodes)

  ▪ Increase in temperature (38°–41°C, 101°–106°F)

  ▪ Small erythematous patches that rapidly increase in size with erythema, warmth, and tenderness of the extremity

  ▪ Painful and enlarged proximal lymph nodes with recurrent chills and fever

 Nursing Alert
Even minor attacks of inflammatory lymphedema cause residual lymphedema that increases total edema in future recurrences.

NURSING ASSESSMENT

- Patient history:
  - Assess for patient history of lymphedema or unexplained swelling of any extremity
    - Date/age at onset
    - Secondary to disease (cancer or infectious), treatment (radiation), or accident or trauma
    - What body parts are affected? (arms, legs, chest, trunk, abdomen, genitalia)
  - Assess family history of lymphedema or unexplained swelling of any extremity
    - Number of relatives with lymphedema
  - Ask patient and caregiver regarding any past surgeries in the affected extremity
    - Reason for surgery
    - Date of surgery
  - Assess pain level
    - What causes the pain?
    - What relieves or reduces the pain?[3]
  - Does the patient have a daily self-management plan for the lymphedema? What is it? Have the patient demonstrate the plan.
    - Bandages
      - Type and number used in 1 year
    - Garments
      - Type and number used in 1 year
      - When and where last fitted
      - Current fit of garments
    - Medications (list these)
    - Manual lymph drainage (when? how often? length of treatment, who performs this if patient is unable to self-manage?)
    - Herbal or alternative medications (list these)

- ■ Yoga, meditation, other alternative treatments (list these)
    - ■ If the patient does not currently follow a self-management plan, assess the rationale for this behavior
  — Assess patient and caregiver knowledge of pathophysiology of lymphedema and related treatment
- Physical Assessment

Signs and symptoms of lymphedema differentiate from venous insufficiency:

  — Tightness and swelling is most often unilateral and symmetrical; venous stasis is most often bilateral and often not symmetrical
  — Joint immobility and pain in the joint exists; often misdiagnosed as arthritis; not present with venous stasis unless the patient also has arthritis
  — Progresses slowly over weeks to months to years; venous stasis often rapid
  — No enlargement of superficial veins exists; may be present in venous stasis
  — Pain occurs during acute cellulitus or lymphangitis
  — Usually no ulcerations present except for cellulitus or lymphangitis
- Long-term effects of lymphedema:
  — Obesity
  — Skin changes: red macular areas, rashes, erythema, cracking, and dryness
  — Minor to severe infections
  — Increased risk of lymphangiosarcoma if lymphedema goes untreated

STAGES OF LYMPHEDEMA

The three stages of lymphedema are:
- Stage I (reversible lymphedema)
  — Swelling of the extremity that usually reduces with elevation
  — Pitting edema (any level of pitting)

- Stage II (spontaneously irreversible lymphedema)
  — Increased fibrous tissue
  — Progressive tissue hardening
  — May cause frequent skin infections
  — Increased edema
  — No pitting of skin even with edema
  — Simple elevation no longer effective to reduce edema
- Stage III (lymphostatic elephantiasis)
  — Elephantiasis nostras verrucosa: progressive histopathologic state characterized by chronic inflammatory fibrosis, epidermal hyperplasia, and hypertrophy of subcutaneous and cutaneous connective tissue.
    - Extreme change in edema
    - Limbs become columnar (knees and ankles lose definition)
    - Increased skin hardening
    - May cause large hanging skin folds
    - May be associated with Stewart-Treves syndrome (highly malignant angiosarcoma)

DIAGNOSIS OF LYMPHEDEMA[7,9,13,14]

Lymphedema is diagnosed by presence of the following:

- Symptomatic patient history
- Presence of symptoms is usually enough to positively diagnose 90% of cases
- CT or MRI of lymph nodes demonstrate edema or fibrosis
- Lymphangiography—x-ray of the lymph system—with injection of oil-based contrast dye is no longer performed as it sometimes damages the remaining functioning lymphatic vessels
- Lymphoscintigraphy—an alternative imaging technique— with injection of water-based dye is now considered safest and most accepted method of diagnostic testing

MANAGEMENT AND TREATMENT[8,12] OF LYMPHEDEMA

* No known cure at this time
* Treatment may delay or prevent disease progression
* Surgery such as lymphovenous shunt (occasionally used for severe cases but not usually treatment of choice)
* Nonsurgical treatments
  — Antibiotics for active infection
  — Antibiotics may also be used prophylactically in individuals with frequent infections
  — Benzopyrones (Coumarin NOT Coumadin); these are not anticoagulants (they are benzopyrones) and are not commonly used in the United States
    ▪ Benzopyrones aid in removing excess protein and therefore reducing edema by causing an increase in macrophages in the area
    ▪ This approach is slow (takes months)
      ○ Educate patients to take oral doses (topical medication not used in US) with food. Side effects include dizziness, drowsiness, nausea, or diarrhea usually in the first month of use.
  — Complex physical decongestive therapy (CPDT), complex physical therapy (CPT), or complex lymphedema therapy (CLT)
  — Four components to these therapies[6,11]
    ▪ Decongestion or manual lymph drainage (MLD): gentle, daily massage and physiotherapy to improve lymph flow
    ▪ Compression therapy to prevent reaccumulation of fluid; done by tightly wrapping limb after each MLD session
    ▪ When maximal reduction in edema is achieved (often after 1 month or longer) patient is fitted with compression garment that requires custom fitting and is often custom-made

- Meticulous skin care to avoid infections
  - Decrease dermal fungal or bacterial colonization that may lead to infections
  - Low pH skin lotions or moisturizers to reduce skin drying and microbial growth
  - Treat immediately any breaks in skin due to impaired local immunity that may lead to infections
- Remedial exercises while wearing compression garments to improve muscle tone and propel flow of lymph

— Compression garments
- Educate patient and caregiver
  - Gaining or losing weight will effect the efficacy of the garment and therefore they should see either health-care provider or individual who fitted the garment
  - Garment must be worn every day (sometimes the patient does not have to wear the garment 24 hours a day; others will wear the garment day and night)
  - Follow manufacturer's instructions regarding washing, drying, and if lotion or cream can be used on the extremity before applying the garment
  - Protect the garment from rings, fingernails, and other items that may snag or tear the fabric
  - Check the garment daily for fit; if it does not fit correctly contact the provider or fitter
  - Amount of exercise that may be performed while wearing the garment
  - Garment should be washed or changed to a fresh garment daily
  - Garment should be replaced according to manufacturer's or provider's recommendation. Therefore keep a calendar of when the garment was purchased and when it was first used.

Nursing Tip
If the garment chafes, is too loose, or is too tight, notify the provider or fitter. If elasticity is lost or the garment is damaged, it must be replaced. Ordering new garments must be done before the old one wears out.

— Avoid injury and seek immediate medical attention should injury occur.[10]
— Educate the patient and caregiver to assess the limb twice a day for pain and swelling and to report symptoms to the provider or fitter
  ▪ Avoid the following injuries:
  ▪ Temperature extremes
  ▪ Burns
  ▪ Insect bites
  ▪ Pet or other scratches
  ▪ Gardening accidents
  ▪ Cuts from nail care. Inform the nail care technician of the risk of infection prior to care. NOTE: health-care providers should approve any nail care and may suggest professional care from someone other than a nail care technician.
— Avoid chemical hair removers. Use only a well maintained electric razor if shaving is necessary and avoid blade razors
— Avoid pounding of high-impact athletic activity
— Daily low-impact exercise is necessary such as walking or swimming with the garment in place
— Elevate the limb during rest and sleep periods
— Keep all skin clean; use a patting, nonvigorous method of drying the skin
— Regularly launder all fabrics that contact the skin

— Use moisturizing lotion following the manufacturer's instructions
— Avoid extreme temperature changes
— Bathing, showering, swimming
— Hot tubs, spas, saunas
— Washing anything (dishes, car, floors, or laundry)
— With therapeutic treatments

- Before starting any exercise program the individual with lymphedema or at risk of lymphedema should have clearance from his or her primary provider.
- Initiate all activities slowly and cautiously and discontinued at any time pain, discomfort, or increased edema occurs.
- Never perform any activity to exhaustion
- Barometric pressure at high altitudes can cause an onset of or exacerbate lymphedema; compression garment must be worn with high-altitude activities such as airplane flying, hiking or biking[2] (at altitudes higher than those in which the individual lives).
- Keep skin dry especially in warm, humid climates; may use cornstarch
- Maintain ideal body weight
- Drink fluids (purified water is best, 2 ounces for every pound of body weight is recommended)
- High-protein diet (unless contraindicated); use easily digestible proteins for 10% to 30% of calorie intake

ADDITIONAL MANAGEMENT OPTIONS

- Lymphedema Pumps
  — Sequential via pneumatic compression device
  — Patient should elevate legs for 30 minutes before applying pump
  — Pumping is usually done twice a day for 2 hours at a time

— Contraindications
  ▪ Cellulitus or infections
  ▪ Acute conditions where fracture may be present
  ▪ Presence of thrombophlebitis
  ▪ Peripheral vascular disease

INTERNET RESOURCES

- **National Lymphedema Network.**
  —http://www.lymphnet.org/
- **Lymphology Association of North America.**
  —http://www.clt-lana.org/
- **International Society of Lymphology.**
  —http://www.u.arizona.edu/~witte/ISL.htm
  —ftp://67305:mcgraw@ftp.inttype.com/Outgoing/Barberio/FirstPages/
- **Children with lymphedema (support group for children and parents).**
  —http://health.groups.yahoo.com/group/childrenwith-lymphedema
- **National Association of Rare Disorders (Primary lymphedema).**
  —http://www.rarediseases.org/
- **The Susan G. Koman Breast Cancer Foundation.**
  —http://cms.komen.org/komen/index.htm

REFERENCES

1. National lymphedema network hhttp://www.lymphnet.org/pdfDocs/nlnexercise.pdfhttp://www.lymphnet.org/pdfDocs/nlnexercise.pdf. Accessed May 12, 2007.
2. Selim S, et al. Living with Lymphedema www.lymphnet.org/pdfDocs/nlnexercise.pdf. Accessed May 12, 2007.

3. Kosir MA, et al. Surgical outcomes after breast cancer surgery: Measuring acute lymphedema. *Journal of Surgical Research.* Feb 2001;95(2):147–151.

4. Ferrell RE, et al. Hereditary lymphedema: evidence for linkage and genetic heterogeneity. *Human Molecular Genetics.* 1998;7:2073–2078.

5. Hinrichs CS, et al. Lymphedema secondary to postmastectomy radiation: Incidence and risk factors. *Annals of Surgical Oncology.* 2004;11:573–580.

6. Korosec BJ. Manual lymphatic drainage therapy. *Home Health Care Management Practice.* Oct 1, 2004;16(6):499–511.

7. Tiwari A, et al. Differential diagnosis, investigation, and current treatment of lower limb lymphedema. *Archives of Surgery.* 2003;138:152–161.

8. Dell DD, et al. Caring for a patient with lymphedema. *Nursing.* June 2006;36(6):49–51.

9. Sander AP, et al. Upper-extremity volume measurements in women with lymphedema: A comparison of measurements obtained via water displacement with geometrically determined volume. *Physical Therapy.* Dec 2002;82(12):1201–1212.

10. Macdonald J. Lymphedema, lipedema, and the open wound. The role of compression therapy. *Surgical Clinics of North America.* 2003;8(3):639–658.

11. Cheville A, et al. Lymphedema management. *Seminars in Radiation Oncology.* 2003;13(3):290–301.

12. Franks PJ, et al. Assessment of health-related quality of life in patients with lymphedema of the lower limb. *Wound Repair and Regeneration.* Mar-Apr 2006;14(2):110–118.

13. Baranoski S, Ayello E. *Wound Care Essentials Practice Principles.* Philadelphia, PA: Lippincott Williams & Wilkins; 2004.

14. Bryant RA. *Acute and Chronic Wounds* 2nd ed. Louis, MO: Mosby; 2000.

SUGGESTED READING

Baranoski S, Ayello E. *Wound Care Essentials Practice Principles.* Philadelphia, PA: Lippincott Williams & Wilkins; 2004.

Bryant RA. *Acute and Chronic Wounds* 2nd ed. Louis, MO: Mosby; 2000.

Ennis WJ, Meneses P. Wound healing at the local level: the stunned wound. *Ostomy/Wound Management*. January 2000;46(suppl 1A): S39–S48.

Falanga V. Wound bed preparation and the role of enzymes: a case for multiple actions of therapeutic agents. *Wounds*. 2002;14(2):47–57.

Hall JC. *Sauer's Manual of Skin Diseases*. 8th ed. Philadelphia, PA: Lippincott Williams & Wilkins; 2000.

Hess CT. *Wound Care*. 2nd ed. Springhouse, PA: Springhouse Corp; 1998.

Hess CT. *Wound Care*. 3rd ed. Springhouse, PA: Springhouse Corp; 2000.

Lopez AP, et al. Venous ulcers. *Wounds*. 1998;10(5):149.

Mahler GD, et al, (eds). *Clinician's Pocket Guide to Chronic Wound Repair*. Springhouse, PA: Springhouse Corp; 1999.

Mertz PM, Ovington LG. Wound healing microbiology. *Dermatology Clinics*. Oct. 1993;11(4):739–747.

Mondary T, Riffenburgh RH, Johnstone PAS. Prospective trial of complete decongestive therapy for upper extremity lymphedema after breast cancer therapy. *The Cancer Journal*. 2004;10(1): 42–48.

Mozes G, et al. A surgical anatomy for endoscopic subfascial division of perforating veins. *Journal of Vascular Surgery*. 1996;24: 800–808.

O'Donnell TF, et al. Chronic venous insufficiency and varicose veins. In: Young JR, et al. *Peripheral Vascular Diseases*. 2nd ed. St. Louis, MO: Mosby; 1996.

O'Donnell TF, et al. Chronic venous insufficiency. In: Jarrett F, et al. *Vascular Surgery of the Lower Extremities*. St. Louis, MO: Mosby; 1996.

Papadopopoulos A, et al. Motivation and compliance in wound management. *Journal of Wound Care*. October 1999;8(9): 467–469.

Patrek JA, Pressman PI, Smith RA. Lymphedema: current issues in research and management. *CA: A Cancer Journal for Clinicians.*, 2000;50(5):292–307.

Petro J. Ethical and psychosocial considerations of wound management. *Decubitus.* January 1992;22–25.

Queral LA, et al. Mini-incisional ligation of incompetent perforating veins of the legs. *Journal of Vascular Surgery.* 1997;25:437–441.

Reichardt LE. Venous ulceration: compression as the mainstay of therapy. *JWOCN.* 1999;26(1):39.

Rhinehart E. Infection control in home care. *Emerg Infect Dis.* 2001;7(2). Available from: .www.medscape.com. Accessed

Scanlon VC, et al. *Essentials of Anatomy and Physiology.* 3rd ed. Philadelphia, PA: FA Davis; 1999;67–99.

Seaman S. Evaluation and management of lower extremity ulcers: adherence to prescribed therapy can save limbs. *Advance for Nurse Practitioners.* March 2002;32–47.

Seidel H, Ball J, Dains J, Benedict GW. *Mosby's Guide to Physical Examination.* 4th ed. St Louis, MO: Mosby Inc; 1999.

Stalano-Coico L, et al. Wound fluids: a reflection of the state of healing. *Ostomy/Wound Management.* January 2000;46 (supplement 1A): S85–S93.

Sussman C, Bates-Jensen B. *Wound Care A Collaborative Practice Manual for Physical Therapists and Nurses.* Gaithersburg, MD: Aspen Publications; 1998.

Swartz M. *Textbook of Physical Diagnosis History and Examination.* 3rd ed. Philadelphia, PA: WB Saunders Co; 1998.

Terry M, et al. Tobacco: its impact on vascular disease. *Surg Clin North Amer.* 1998;78(3):409.

Tierney L, McPhee S, Papadakis M. *Current Medical Diagnosis and Treatment.* 37th ed. Stamford, CT: Appleton & Lange; 1998.

Tiwari A, Koon-Sung C, Button M, Myint Fl, Hamilton G, Differential diagnosis, investigation, and current treatment of lower limb lymphedema. *Archives of Surgery.* 2003;138(2): 152–161.

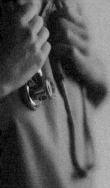

Chapter 8

ASSESSMENT OF OTHER WOUND TYPES

KEY POINTS

- Cutaneous Metastases: Etiology, Treatment, and Management
- Burns: Types, Assessment, and Management
- Atypical Wounds: Assessment and Management

CUTANEOUS METASTASES[1,2]

Etiology:

- Occur in 2.7% to 4.4% of all cancer patients[1]
- May present as the initial sign of cancer, after discovery of the primary cancer, or late in the course of the disease.
- Most commonly associated with advanced systemic disease
- Expected survival is less than 1 year
- Occurs most frequently in:
  — Women with breast cancer (18.6% to 50%)[1]
  — Men with bronchogenic carcinoma (3% to 7.5%)[1]
- Melanoma, oral cavity, renal, colon, and gastric primary cancers cause 90% of all cutaneous metastases in patients with these cancers.[1]
- Cutaneous lesions may also be caused by Kaposi sarcoma, lymphoma, and leukemia.
- Occurrence of cutaneous metastases is a result of:
  — Primary tumor proliferation
  — Local extension
    - Vascular and/or lymphatic penetration and embolization
    - Release of malignant cells for transport to distant sites and/or accidental mechanical implantation of malignant cells during diagnostic or operative procedures.

Appearance

- Cutaneous metastases vary widely and can be misdiagnosed or mistaken for benign skin alterations.

- Often develops as:
  - — Hard, nonmovable nodules
  - — Plaque formations
  - — Ulcerating wounds
- Diagnosis is based on:
  - — Clinical findings
  - — Histopathology (biopsy taken from nonnecrotic areas including a sample of adjacent, noninvolved tissue for comparison)
  - — Location
  - — Distribution
  - — Configuration
  - — Size
  - — Morphological structure (nodule, scale, crust, erosion, fissure)
  - — Drainage (color, amount, character)
  - — Odor of lesion

Location

- Most common location is on the anterior trunk
- Other sites are head, neck, posterior trunk, flanks, and pelvis
- Rarely affects the extremities (these are usually melanomas)

Characteristics

- Tumor invasion with rupture of capillaries
- Necrosis and infection
- Friable tissue which is often purulent and odorous

Treatment and Management

- Dependent on the stage of the disease
- Primary management is to treat the underlying malignancy
  - — Use systemic therapy with or without local treatment

- Solitary lesions require:
  — Surgical excision
  — Irradiation
  — Local or systemic chemotherapy
  — Hormones
  — Immunotherapy
- Multiple lesions require:
  — Systemic chemotherapy
  — Palliative treatment used in advanced disease and advanced lesions
- Goals of secondary or palliative management:
  — Minimize potential complications
    - Infection
    - Bleeding/trauma
    - Odor
    - Pain
    - Social ostracism/isolation (due to visible lesions and/or odor)
  — Minimize bleeding related to trauma:
    - Avoid physical irritants
    - Shear
    - Friction
    - Pressure
  — Use extreme gentleness with all dressing changes/treatments of affected areas
  — Avoid temperature extremes
  — Avoid chemical irritants
    - Body secretions
    - Medications
    - Body excretions
    - Most soaps, lotions
    - Extra care with wound cleansing if necessary

- Control bleeding
  - Anticoagulant dressings (surgical absorbable dressings)
    - Hemostat/Gelfoam, Surgicel (Johnson & Johnson)
    - $AgNO_3$ (silver nitrate cautery) for local bleeding sites ONLY; requires procedure and policy
  - Change dressing ONLY with strike-through or leakage, as needed
- Prevent infection
  - Physical barrier on ulcerated lesions to prevent contamination
  - Aseptic technique with all dressing changes/treatment
  - Absorbable dressings
    - Hydrocolloid (early stages with little exudate)
    - Hydrogel sheets (early stages with little exudate)
    - Hydrophilic beads/powders
    - Cotton dressings
- Treat infection
  - Culture for aerobic and anaerobic organisms
    - Topical organism specific antibiotics: powders are better than ointments
    - Systemic antibiotics organism specific
  - Change dressing at least daily
- Odor management
  - Remove necrotic tissue
  - Clean with povidone-iodine or weak Dakin's solution (less than 1/4 strength) or weak acetic acid solution (less than 0.25%)
  - Apply baking soda in between dressing layers
  - Use air fresheners or odor eliminators such as room deodorizers
  - Cleanse with one of the above cleansers, rinse with normal saline, apply plain yogurt or buttermilk to lesion, leave on for 15 to 20 minutes, irrigate off with normal saline, and apply dressing
  - On secondary (outer) dressing apply Balsam of Peru in a grid-like fashion

— Place a shallow pan of activated charcoal one-quarter inch thick in patient's room, change every 3 to 5 days
— Apply gauze saturated with Cepacol for 15 to 20 minutes, rinse with normal saline, and apply dressing
— Apply odor-controlling charcoal dressings
— Apply antibiotic/antifungal agents topically or systemically
— Refer to wound, ostomy, continence nurse (WOCN) especially if custom made, fitted wound, or ostomy collection devices may be necessary

- Debridement
  — Use with caution as it may cause bleeding or erosion
  — Mechanical irrigation with 19 g catheter and 30 cc syringe
  — Mechanical jet/pulsed lavage
  — Whirlpool
  — Wet-to-dry dressings (allow to dry then lift off at 90 degree angle)
  — Hydrocolloid dressings/transparent adhesive dressings
  — Half-strength hydrogen peroxide
  — Burrow solution (aluminum acetate)
  — Dakin's solution (sodium hypochlorite)
  — Debridement enzymes such as Santyl and Accuzyme

- Psychosocial Care
  — Intensify professional vigilance in screening for psychological distress and psychiatric disorders
    - Social isolation
    - Despair
    - Avoidance

BURNS

Types of burns

- Thermal burns
  — Heat is transferred to the body through conduction, radiation, and convection.

■ Most common is conduction; direct contact of the body to some heat source such as boiling liquid.

■ Radiation is a process of kinetic energy being concerted to electromagnetic energy, which then travels through space until contacting an object at which time it is again converted to kinetic energy. Trauma is caused by the energy transfer such as in tanning beds and heat lamps.

■ Convection utilizes air currents which carry the heat such as an explosion that causes flash injuries.

— Depth of thermal injury determined by:

■ Temperature to which the tissue is heated

■ Duration of the exposure to the elevated temperature

  ○ As exposure temperatures increase a variety of cellular functions become impaired.

   • 40° to 44°C (104° to 110°F) inhibits cellular enzymatic reactions and failure of membrane sodium pump follows which results in increased intracellular sodium levels.

   • 60°C (140°F) exposure for 1 second causes epidermal sloughing which results in partial thickness loss.

   • 70°C (158°F) denatures dermal protein results in full thickness loss.

• Chemical burns

— Noxious substances that come in contact with the skin thereby causing tissue damage or reaction.

■ Amount of tissue damage depends on concentration and quality of noxious substance

■ Total length of time of exposure

■ Mechanism of chemical action

■ These agents generally continue to cause damage until they are deactivated by:

  ○ Local tissue reaction

  ○ External agent neutralization

  ○ Dilution by water

■ All these agents cause protein coagulation either through principles of oxidizing, reduction, corrosion, desiccation, or as vesicants.

  ○ Oxidizing: inserts an oxygen atom into a protein thereby inhibiting the protein's normal function.

  ○ Reduction: denature protein by reducing the amide links between proteins (this reduction may create heat and therefore these injuries may be a combination of thermal and chemical).

  ○ Corrosion: denature protein but the exact mechanism of this is depends on the chemical agent.

  ○ Desiccation: extract water from the tissues which may also initiate an exothermic reaction that causes thermal as well as chemical injury.

  ○ Vessicants: cause damage to the DNA and therefore the cells cannot reproduce.

  ○ Chemical agents also cause systemic effects from inhalation and cutaneous absorption.

- Electrical burns:

  — Joule law: quantity of heat produced by an electrical current (J) is directly proportional to the square of the voltage of the current (I) multiplied by the resistance of the conductor (R) and the duration of the contact (T). This injury therefore depends on:

    ■ Type of current encountered
    ■ Pathway of the current flow
    ■ Local tissue resistance
    ■ Duration of the contact

  — The electrical current will follow the closest path through the body from the contact point to the ground where there is the least resistance.

    ■ The more resistant the tissue the greater the heat that is produced as the current passes through.

    ■ Amount of skin resistance possible during the passing of the current is determined by:

- Thickness
- Cleanliness
- Wetness

(Lowest resistance where skin is thin, clean, and wet)

— Amount of skin damage is always deceptively small compared to damage to the internal muscle, fat, and fascia.
— Broad classification of electrical injury:
  - True electrical injury: electricity passes through the body after contact with some type of conductor.
    - Classic entrance and exit wounds and significant deep tissue destruction.
    - Exit wound generally where victim was grounded and most often is larger in size than the contact point entrance wound.
  - Arc burn: caused when an electrical current that is flowing external to the body jumps from the contact point to the ground point. Most often associated with high-tension current.
    - May have entry and exit wound but more common to have scattered areas or spots of injury where the current momentarily contacted the body before jumping to the ground.
    - Tetanic muscle contractions are an acute complication especially with high voltage injury.
    - Fractures, dislocations, intraperitoneal damage, cardiac dysfunctions are often seen.
    - Delayed neurologic changes and cataracts may also occur.
- Radiation burns:
  - Most frequent cause is exposure to ionizing radiation from a local accident or secondary to radiation therapy treatment.
    - Damage to tissues is caused by transference of radiant energy to the body which is then stimulated to form free radicals (highly reactive chemical products).

o These products then form cellular toxins and cause intracellular and molecular damage; cells that divide most rapidly are the most susceptible to damage (skin, bone marrow, GI tract).

Patient Assessment

- Requires total body systems evaluation at each visit if burn is of any significance.
  - — Neurologic/neurogenic: burn patients often experience constant, chronic background pain.
    - ■ Treatments often initiate acute pain
    - ■ Anxiety increases the hyperalgesia of the burn and also often alters pain behaviors
  - — Metabolic: burn patients generally prefer ambient temperatures of about 32°C (90°F)
  - — Sleep disturbances: hospital stays often interrupt normal sleep-wake times as well as bowel evacuation. Sleep may be disturbed by nightmares. Daytime anxiety is also often seen. Many patients suffer from post-traumatic stress disorder (PTSD).
  - — Cardiovascular: cardiovascular function is disrupted whenever 40% or more of the total body surface area (TBSA) has been involved.
    - ■ Edema
    - ■ Depression of cardiac output (most often in the acute phase)
  - — Pulmonary: left-sided heart failure may occur as well as pulmonary edema. Patient may also have experienced respiratory failure while in the hospital as well as adult respiratory distress syndrome (ARDS).
  - — Gastrointestinal: altered nutrient processing requires that the patient consistently receive adequate nutrition throughout the recovery.
    - ■ During the acute phase the body may become stripped of its nutritional stores.

- Decreases in intestinal motility are not uncommon with resultant reduction in absorption as well as peristalsis. The burn patient may have experienced a paralytic ileus in the acute setting.
- The intestinal bacterial barrier is also often compromised during the acute phase of treatment. This failure may result in bacterial translocation and thereby cause systemic sepsis and/or multiple organ dysfunction syndrome (MPDS).

— Hematopoietic: burn patients may have significant losses of red blood cells with resultant hypoxia during the early treatment of the injuries.
- The circulating levels of iron are also depressed after a burn injury. These events may trigger the body to increase erythrocyte production.
- Bone marrow stores are often depleted during the early phases of treatment.
- Platelets may also be depleted in the early phase of treatment.
- Many burn victims have received transfusions of one or more blood components during the acute phase of treatment and may be experiencing anxiety concerning this.

— Renal: renal failure is not uncommon during the early phase of treatment.

— Immunologic: during the treatment burn patients commonly undergo profound immunologic changes.
- Frequent problems are infections caused by gram negative organisms as well as by fungi.

— Long-term physiologic sequelae:
- Height/weight gain delays
- Decreased bone density
- Increased fracture rates
- Temporary menses cessation
- Increased potential for spontaneous abortion or premature parturition

- Abnormal lung function (45% incidence more than 2 years after injury)
- Increased dead space/tidal volume ratio (up to 2.5 years after inhalation injury)
- Children with burns often fail to "catch-up" in growth relative to normal age-related growth.

Burn Management

- Requires a multidisciplinary management strategy and carefully choreographed plan of care
  - Wound care may be provided by the nurse, family member, or patient
    - Pain control
    - Odor control
  - Exudate containment
  - Infection prevention/treatment
  - Graft care
  - Debridement
  - Dressings: ideal properties
    - Absence of antigenicity
    - Tissue compatibility
    - Absence of local or systemic toxicity
    - Water vapor transmission similar to normal skin
    - Impermeability to exogenous microorganisms
    - Rapid and sustained adherence to wound surface
    - Inner surface structure permits ingrowth of fibrovascular tissue
    - Flexibility and pliability that permits conformation to irregular wound surfaces
    - Resistance to linear and shear stresses
    - Prevention of wound surface flora proliferation and reduction of bacterial density

- ■ Tensile strength that resists fragmentation and retention of membrane fragments with removal
- ■ Biodegradability (except for permanently implanted membranes)
- ■ Low cost
- ■ Indefinite shelf life
- ■ Minimal storage requirements
- Contracture and scar management
- PT/OT/SLP
- Medical social worker: long-term plan, vocational rehabilitation, financial planning
- Chaplain
- CHHA: home rehabilitation plan, restorative nursing plan
- Supplies and DME coordination

Irradiated Skin Management

- All of the above for burn management as appropriate
- Prevent trauma to skin that has been irradiated
  - — No soap or mildest soap use only
  - — Rinse soap thoroughly
  - — Pat skin dry with soft, cotton, absorbent material; do NOT rub skin
  - — No bathing or soaking in hot water
  - — Do not use detergent soaps or bubble bath in bathing water
  - — No perfumes, deodorants, or makeup on irradiated skin during treatment and only as needed after treatment is completed (some patients may never be able to use these product types)
  - — No tight fitting clothing in the treatment field during treatment and as above as needed
  - — No heating devices or ice packs or cooling devices on irradiated areas

— No sun exposure to irradiated area; utilize sun block (after treatment completed), cover treated area with soft, cotton material; use umbrellas, hats, etc.

— Microporous adhesives only in treated area, use skin barrier wipe under adhesives after patch testing

— No scratching of treated skin

— Lotions or moisturizers that are approved by radiation therapy specialist during treatment and only after patch testing after treatments are completed

  ▪ Aquaphor and Biafine are commonly allowed products

Care for Radiation-Damaged Skin

• Hydrogel wafer or sheet to reddended areas for comfort and pain reduction. Avoid maceration.

• Nonadhesive dressings only in the skin fold during treatment, verify appropriateness with radiation specialist before treatment.

• Exudative skin

  — Foam

  — Alginate

  — Impregnated gauze

  — Notify radiation therapy physician of skin condition as soon as condition is detected.

Hyperbaric Oxygen

Definition: "the delivery of oxygen at pressure greater than 1 atmosphere (atm), is a form of therapy capable of inducing revascularization of damaged tissue."[4]

• Two types of hyperbaric oxygen:

  — Systemic: patient is placed in a chamber where pure oxygen is breathed at increased atmospheric pressures.

  — Topical: patient's limb is enclosed in a container such as a plastic bag and oxygen is applied locally.

- Effects of hyberbaric oxygen (HBO):
  - Increased pressure creates a mechanical effect. Volume of any trapped free gas in the body will decrease as increasing pressure is exerted on it. This causes a reduction of bubble size and may enable it to pass through the circulation or travel to a smaller vessel where it results in a smaller area of infarction. This is used for management of gas embolism and decompression sickness.
  - When the body is flooded with oxygen, other gases are forced out thereby reducing toxic effects of gases such as carbon monoxide.
  - HBO functions like an alpha-adrenergic drug causing vasoconstriction and is used in crush injuries or to reduce the edema of burns.
  - HBO creates an environment in which anaerobes cannot survive as these bacteria do not have natural defenses to protect them from superoxides or peroxides, which are formed in the presence of high oxygen tensions. Other body bacterial defenses (i.e., phagocytic leukocytes) in the body are oxygen dependent and HBO creates a reoxygenation that enhances their activity.
  - Extra oxygen is physically dissolved into the plasma and therefore in ischemic conditions the quantity of oxygen carried and transferred to the tissue is increased. This oxygen excess allows tissues to meet increased metabolic needs for healing.

- Indications for HBO:
  - Air or gas embolism
  - Carbon monoxide poisoning
  - Crush injury, compartment syndrome, and acute traumatic ischemias
  - Cyanide poisoning
  - Decompression sickness

— Specific refractory anaerobic infections
— Exceptional blood loss
— Anemia
— Gas gangrene
— Necrotizing soft tissue infections such as fasciitis
— Refractory osteomyelitis: to cause neovascularization of ischemic bone
— Radiation necrosis
— Thermal burns and scalds
— Specific wounds as an enhancement of healing:
  ▪ Pyoderma gangrenosum
  ▪ Diabetic foot and leg ulcers
  ▪ Traumatic ischemic lesions
  ▪ Varicose ulceration
  ▪ Clostridial infections
• Patient adherence to treatment regimen is required:
— Stop smoking
— Follow-up treatments
— Wound care
— Appropriate nutrition

ATYPICAL WOUNDS: PATHOPHYSIOLOGY AND MANAGEMENT

Vasculitis

• Group of disorders with the pathologic feature of vascular inflammation and necrosis
• Vasculitides is the broad term reflecting the systemic disorders that cause vasculitis
— Affects vessels of any type
— Any organ or body system may be involved
— Various symptoms and clinical presentations

— The wounds are generally a sign of a complex process
— The wound may indicate a systemic disorder
— Pathogenesis, in part, is immunologic
  ▪ Various immune complexes are deposited on vessel walls. This causes leukocyte infiltration and release of various enzymes resulting in necrosis to the vessel wall.
  ▪ The categories of vasculitis reflect the size of the vessels involved, small, medium, or large.
— Specific diseases that may contribute or cause ulcers:
  ▪ Rheumatoid arthritis
  ▪ System lupus erythematosus
  ▪ Polyarteritis nodosa
  ▪ Hypersensitivity vasculitis
  ▪ Wegener granulomatosis (respiratory involvement possible)
  ▪ Sjogren syndrome (oral and ocular dryness)
  ▪ Cryoglobulinemic vasculitis (renal and skin problems)
  ▪ Dermatomyositis
— Signs and symptoms:
  ▪ Fever
  ▪ Myalgias
  ▪ Arthralgias
  ▪ Malaise
  ▪ Vague, flu-like illness may be reported
  ▪ Common cutaneous features
    ○ Erythematous macules and nodules to hemorrhagic vessels
    ○ Palpable purpura to necrotic lesions and ulcerations
    ○ Location: frequently on lower extremities near malleoli
  ▪ Other symptoms are dependent on the organ involved and the specific disease

- Treatment
  - Biopsy (best when taken from early purpuric lesions)
    - 2 to 3 sites may be necessary for diagnosis
  - Control underlying disease
  - Steroids
  - Immunosuppressive therapy
  - Plasmapheresis in severe cases to remove circulating immune complexes
  - Topical treatment
    - Debridement of necrotic and devitalized tissue
    - Identification and treatment of infection
    - Moist wound bed
    - Absorption of excess exudate
    - Pack dead space
    - Insulate and protect from additional trauma
    - Topical application vitamin A to counteract steroid therapy antiinflammatory effects

Rheumatoid Arthritis

- High levels of rheumatoid factor
- Rheumatoid nodules typically on hands and elbows
- Venous insufficiency symptoms
  - Decreased ankle movement leads to poor calf muscle pump function that increases patient risk for developing venous ulcers
- Initially palpable purpura and ecchymosis which may progress to ulceration
  - Shallow, well demarcated, painful
  - Slow to heal
- Compression therapy may be necessary if the limb is edematous from venous insufficiency

Systemic Lupus Erythematosus (SLE)

- Occurs primarily in young women 10 to 50 years[5]
- African Americans and Asians are affected more often than people from other races.[5]
- Approximately 70% have some form of skin disease
- Triggering factors
  — Sunlight and medications (procainamide and hydralazine hydrochloride, [Apresoline])
- Photosensitivity common
- Oral ulcers also common
- Erythematous, scaly lesions which may occur then appear to resolve
- Palpable purpura that may progress to ulceration
- Malleolar region common location
- Round lesions with erythematous borders
- Ulceration may atrophy and have loss of pigmentation

Polyarteritis Nodosa (PAN)

- Approximately 40% of individuals have skin involvement
- Punched out lesions
- Painful
- Initially may present as purpura with urticaria and then progress to ulceration
- Starburst pattern may extend from ulcer
- Subcutaneous, painful nodules also present

Hypersensitivity Vasculitis

- Approximately 50% is idiopathic
- Associated with hypersensitivity to antigens from infectious agents (e.g., group A streptococci, hepatitis B virus, etc.), drugs (penicillin, sulfonamides, serums) or endogenous

(systemic lupus erythematous, rheumatoid arthritis, carcinoma of kidney) or other exogenous sources.

- Small vessel (primarily venules) involvement
- Segmental inflammation and fibrinoid necrosis
- May have pruritis, burning pain, or no symptoms
- ESR often elevated
- Urinalysis may show red blood cell casts and albuminuria
- Lesions:
  — Palpable purpura may change to hemorrhagic blisters becoming necrotic and then ulcerating
  — Petechiae: macular (not palpable) or papular petechiae that will be palpable
  — Urticarial wheals (persists longer than 24 hours indicates urticarial vasculitis)
  — Shape: may be round, oval, annular, or arciform that are arranged in various patterns such as scattered, discrete lesions to dense and confluent ones
  — Usually on lower third of legs, ankles, buttocks, or arms
  — Stasis precipitates and aggravates lesions

Wegener Granulomatosis

- Occurs at any age, mean age is 40 years
- Slightly more common in males
- Rare in African Americans
- Approximately 15% of cases develop glomerulitis
- Paranasal sinus pain and purulent or bloody nasal discharge are also symptoms
- Cough, hemoptysis, dyspnea, and chest discomfort are respiratory symptoms
- 45% of patients will develop skin lesions during the course of this condition with 13% demonstrating symptoms initially
- 65% develop mild conjunctivitis

- 85% develop renal failure in advanced disease
  - Fatal due to rapidly progressive renal failure unless treated
- Ulcerations resemble pyoderma grangrenosum
  - Papules, vesicles, and palpable purpura similar to hypersensitivity vasculitis
  - Subcutaneous nodules, plaques, and noduloulcerative lesions similar to PAN
  - Most common on lower extremities; also on face, trunk, and upper extremities
  - Oral ulcerations often first symptom

Cryoglobulinemic Vasculitis

- Less than 50% have cold sensitivity
- Chills, fever, and dyspnea following cold exposure
- Diarrhea following cold exposure
- Arthralgia, renal, neurologic symptoms
- Abdominal pain
- Arterial thrombosis
- Noninflammatory purpura in cold exposed areas
- Inflammatory purpura (may or may not be palpable)
- Purpura following long periods of sitting or standing
- Livedo reticularis on extremities
- Raynaud phenomenon with or without severe resultant finger and toe tip gangrene
- Purpura on lower extremities extending to thighs including the abdomen
- Hemorrhagic necrosis and ulceration on the nose, ears, fingers, and toes

Dermatomyositis

- Occurs in juveniles 5-15 years[6] and adults 40 to 60[6] years

- In individuals older than 55 years often associated with malignancy (tumors of breast, ovary, uterus, lung, stomach, and colon)
- Increased creatinine phosphokinase (65% of patients)
- Increased 24-hour urine creatinine excretion (greater than 200 mg/24h)
- EMG leads to increased irritability
- Progressive muscle weakness with intact deep tendon reflexes
- Difficulty in:
  — Rising from supine position
  — Climbing stairs
  — Raising arms over head
  — Turning in bed
- Dysphagia
- Facial lesions are heliotrope (violet color)
- Other ulcerations and lesions:
  — Papular dermatitis with varying erythema and scaling
  — May become erosions and ulcers; healing with stellate, bizarre scarring
  — Flat-topped, violaceous papules with varying atrophy
  — Periungual erythema and telangiectasia
  — Pressure point distribution especially elbows and knuckles
  — Other distribution on forehead, scalp, neck, and upper chest

Other Atypical Wounds

Pyoderma gangrenosum
- Often misdiagnosed as an infection
- 50% seen in association with:
  — Crohn disease
  — Ulcerative colitis

- — Reumatoid arthritis
- — Monoclonal gammapathy
- — Diverticulitis
- — Arthritis
- — Myeloma
- — Leukemia
- — Active chronic hepatitis
- CBS and ESR may or may not be elevated
- Untreated lasts months to years
- Acute onset often with (usually solitary):
  - — Hemorrhagic pustule
  - — Painful nodule (may or may not follow trauma)
  - — Breakdown of either of the above results in:
    - Ulcer with irregular and raised borders
    - Undermined boggy areas that often drain pus
  - — Ulcer bed is purulent, hemorrhagic, partially covered with eschar with or without granulation tissue
  - — Pustules are often seen at the borders
  - — Borders are dusky red or purple with erythematous halo spreading centrifugally
  - — Healing results in thin, atrophic, cribiform scar
  - — Slight trauma causes new lesions
  - — Common sites
    - Lower extremities
    - Buttocks
    - Abdomen
    - Face

Pemphigus vulgaris (PV)

- Affects individuals aged 40 to 60 years
- Equal in males or females
- Autoimmune disorder, acute or chronic, bullous

- Usually starts orally and months may elapse before skin lesions occur
  — Skin lesions may be localized for 6 to 12 months before generalized bullae occur; less commonly the disease begins with spontaneous generalize bullae eruption
- Epistaxis, hoarseness, and dysphagia occur
- Skin lesions
  — Vesicles to bullae, easily ruptured and weeping
  — Extensive erosions that bleed easily
  — Crusts (particularly on scalp)
- Skin-colored
- Round or oval
- Randomly scattered or discrete lesions
- Pressure on a bulla leads to lateral extension
- Dislodging of epidermis by lateral finger pressure in the vicinity of lesion causes an erosion
- Common sites
  — Scalp
  — Face
  — Chest
  — Axilla
  — Groin
  — Umbilicus
- Treatment is immunosuppressive therapy and concomitant corticosteroids

Bullous pemphigoid

- Autoimmune disorder which presents with chronic bullous eruption
- More common in individuals aged 60 to 80 years than PV
- Equal incidence of males and females
- May start with urticarial lesion that evolves into bullae over weeks or months or occur spontaneously as a generalized eruption
- Eosinophilia

- Skin lesions
  — Erosions
  — Erythematous, urticarial lesions may precede bullae formation by months
  — Bullae are oval or round, large, tense, firm-topped may arise on normal or erythematous skin
  — Arranged in arciform, annular, or serpiginous lesions scattered or discrete
  — Common sites
    - Axillae
    - Medial aspects of thighs
    - Groin
    - Abdomen
    - Flexor aspects of forearms
    - Lower legs (often first manifestation)
    - Mucous membranes
    - Mouth
    - Anus
    - Vagina
  — Treatment
    - Systemic prednisone alone or in combination with azathioprine 150 mg daily for remission (usually seen in a few weeks) then 50 mg to 100 mg per day for maintenance
    - Intralesional corticosteroids may be necessary
    - Topical corticosteroid in mild cases
    - Tetracycline with or without nicotinamide possibly effective

REFERENCES

1. Available at, http://www.deroyal.com/Wound_Care. Accessed January 15, 2008.
2. National Cancer Institute. Available at: http://imsdd.meb.uni-bonn.de/cancernet/304277.html. Accessed March 5, 2007.

3. Pruitt BA, Levine NS. Characteristics and uses of biologic dressings as skin substitutes. *Arch Surg.* 1984;119(3):12–322.

4. McWhorter JW. Hyperbaric oxygen in wound healing. In: McCulloch JM, Kloth LC, Feedar JA (eds). *Wound Healing Alternatives in Management.* 2nd ed. Philadelphia, PA: FA Davis Company; 1995:405–414.

5. National Institute of Health. Available at http://www.nlm.nih.gov/medlineplus/ency/article/000435.htm. Accessed January 10, 2008.

6. National Institute of Health. Available at: http://www.nlm.nih.gov/medlineplus/ency/article/000435.htm. Accessed January 10, 2008.

SUGGESTED READING

Baranoski S, Ayello E. *Wound Care Essentials Practice Principles.* Philadelphia, PA: Lippincott Williams & Wilkins; 2004.

Bryant RA. *Acute and Chronic Wounds.* 2nd ed. Louis, MO: Mosby; 2000.

Cuzzell J. Clues: bruised, torn skin. *AJN.* Mar 1990;16-17.

Ennis WJ, Meneses P. Wound healing at the local level: the stunned wound. *Ostomy/Wound Management.* Jan 2000;46(suppl 1A): S39–S48.

Falanga V. Wound bed preparation and the role of enzymes: a case for multiple actions of therapeutic agents. *Wounds.* 2002;14(2): 47–57.

Hall JC. *Sauer's Manual of Skin Diseases.* 8th ed. Philadelphia, PA: Lippincott Williams & Wilkins; 2000.

Hess CT. *Wound Care.* 2nd ed. Springhouse, PA: Springhouse Corp; 1998.

Hess CT. *Wound Care.* 3rd ed. Springhouse, PA: Springhouse Corp; 2000.

Mahler GD, et al. *Clinician's Pocket Guide to Chronic Wound Repair.* Springhouse, PA: Springhouse Corp; 1999.

Mertz PM, Ovington LG. Wound healing microbiology. *Dermatology Clinics.* Oct 1993;11(4):739–747.

National Cancer Institute. Types of Cancer and Treatment. Available at: http://imsdd.meb.uni-bonn.de/cancernet/304277.html. Accessed March 5, 2007.

Papadopopoulos A, et al. Motivation and compliance in wound management. *Journal of Wound Care*. Oct 1999;8(9):467–469.

Payne RL, et al. Defining and classifying skin tears: need for a common language. *Ostomy/Wound Management*. 1993;39(5):16–26.

Petro J. Ethical and psychosocial considerations of wound management. *Decubitus*. Jan 1992;(4):22–25.

Queral LA, et al. Mini-incisional ligation of incompetent perforating veins of the legs. *Journal of Vascular Surgery*. 1997;25:437–441.

Rhinehart E. Infection control in home care. *Emer Infec Dis*. 2001;7(2):1–12. Available at: www.medscape.com

Scanlon VC, et al. *Essentials of Anatomy and Physiology*. 3rd ed. Philadelphia, PA: FA Davis Co; 1999.

Seidel H, Ball J, Dains J, Benedict GW. *Mosby's Guide to Physical Examination*. 4th ed. St. Louis MO: Mosby Inc; 1999.

Stalano-Coico L, et al. Wound fluids: a reflection of the state of healing. *Ostomy/Wound Management*. Jan 2000;46(suppl 1A):S85–S93.

Sussman C, Bates-Jensen B. *Wound Care A Collaborative Practice Manual for Physical Therapists and Nurses*. Gaithersburg, MD: Aspen Publications; 1998.

Support Systems International, Inc. *The Skin, Module 1*. Charleston, SC: Hillenbrand; 1993.

Swartz M. *Textbook of Physical Diagnosis History and Examination*. 3rd ed. Philadelphia, PA: WB Saunders Co; 1998.

Terry M, et al. Tobacco: its impact on vascular disease. *Surg Clin North Amer*. 1998;78(3):409.

Tierney L, McPhee S, Papadakis M. *Current Medical Diagnosis and Treatment*. 37th ed. Stamford, CT: Appleton & Lange;1998.

Verhaeghe R. Epidemiology and prognosis of peripheral obliterative arteriopathy. *Drugs*. 1998;56(suppl3):1.

White MW, et al. Skin tears in frail elders: a practical approach to prevention. *Geriatric Nursing*. 1994;15(2):95–99.

WOCN Guidance on OASIS Skin and Wound Status MO Items.Spring 2001.

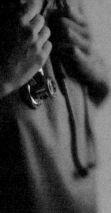

Chapter 9

WOUND MANAGEMENT, PRODUCTS, AND SUPPORT SURFACE SELECTION

KEY POINTS

- Evaluation,
- Diagnosis,
- Goals and Outcomes

EVALUATION

- Evaluation is the assessment and analysis of the findings of:
  — The wound
  — The client physically, mentally, psychosocially, and spiritually
    - Is the client able to learn to perform the necessary care of the wound?
    - Has the client ever provided care to a wound?
  — The caregiver physically, mentally, psychosocially, and spiritually
    - Is the caregiver able to learn to perform the necessary care of the wound?
    - Has the caregiver ever provided care to a wound?
  — If the client is to be discharged to or treated at home. The home environment evaluation includes:
    - Safety? Appropriateness of supplies storage?
    - The ability of the agency and practitioner to manage the wound, patient, caregiver, and environment.
  — If the client is to be discharged to an assisted living or skilled nursing facility
    - What are the applicable laws and ordinances for the specific facility relative to the type of wounds for which care may be safely provided?
      ○ Is the facility able to provide the level of care, the type of wound care, and the frequency of wound care required?

○ What caregiver support will the client be able to receive while in this specific facility (some facilities are too far away for the client's caregiver to travel to in a consistent manner).

DIAGNOSIS

• Judgments, decisions, and conclusions made after the evaluation process is completed about the meaning of the data collected:

— Is the management of the client, wound, caregiver, and environment outside the knowledge, experience, or expertise of the practitioner? If yes, the patient should be referred to the appropriate practitioner.

— This does NOT mean that the practitioner can abandon the patient until the appropriate practitioner is found.

— Must include identifying the disease, condition, or human response from the scientific evaluation of signs, symptoms, history, and diagnostic studies.

— This does NOT mean passive acceptance of the diagnosis that is on the intake or referral form or relying solely on the physician's diagnosis.

▪ In the acute setting, it is the responsibility of the admitting RN to thoroughly evaluate the client and the wound and to collaborate with the attending physician on the diagnosis and the plan of care (POC).

— In the home environment or skilled nursing home in some locations, the diagnosis may be initiated by either the physical therapist or the registered nurse and developed in the terms of that discipline.

— Physical therapists (PT) and registered nurses (RN) may utilize functional diagnoses—assessment of the related impairments and associated disability states that affect both the wound and its ability to heal. Remember that through MDS and OASIS Medicare has mandated that a functional outcome prediction be established at the start of care by the PT/RN.

- Impaired lower/upper extremity strength and/or ROM (manual muscle test) resulting in persistent pressure to the ischial tuberosities.
- Unable to detect pressure or light touch resulting in impaired sensation.
- Chronic inflammation phase resulting in impaired healing.

— RNs may utilize nursing diagnosis using North American Nursing Diagnosis Association list of approved diagnoses. Remember that through MDS and OASIS Medicare has mandated that a functional outcome prediction be established at the start of care.

- Impaired or altered skin integrity r/t immobility and lack of pressure relief or reduction
- Activity intolerance, high risk for altered skin integrity
- Ineffective management of therapeutic regimen

— Remember, the purpose of the diagnosis is to guide in the determination of the most appropriate intervention strategy for the specific patient and NOT because the treatment has worked on some past patients.

- Wound healing phase diagnosis will describe the biologic process of repair that is evaluated from the wound examination.

— In visit and/or treatment documentation the utilization of this will describe the current status of the wound. This also provides a more scientific basis for predicting how the wound healing should proceed or progress.

— 12 possible diagnoses:

1. Chronic inflammation
2. Inflammation
3. Absence of inflammation
4. Chronic proliferation
5. Proliferation

6. Absence of proliferation
7. Chronic epithelialization
8. Epithelialization
9. Absence of epithelialization
10. Chronic remodeling
11. Remodeling
12. Absence of remodeling

— In most wounds these phases are seen in transition and may therefore be documented by describing the dominant phase and the recessive phase such as inflammation; proliferation indicates that the dominant phase is inflammation.

— When two phases seem to dominate, both phases are documented with capital letters as in INFLAMMATION/ PROLIFERATION.

GOALS AND OUTCOMES

• This is the time when the practitioner predicts or develops a prognosis for each specific wound. Prognosis is the maximal improvement expected from an intervention and how long it is expected to take until the wound either reaches the next level of healing, is healed, or is determined to be a chronic wound or one that will not resolve.

• Possible prognoses include:

— Completely healed wound or ideally healed closure; complete wound closure AND successful, functional scar tissue has organized (this is ideal).

— Acceptably closed wound or acceptably healed closure; indicates the wound has resurfaced epithelium that is capable of sustaining functional integrity with ADLs.

— Minimally closed wound or minimally healed closure; reepithelialization has occurred but the wound has not achieved sustained functional integrity and therefore may recur.

— Phase change in the wound. State this as indicated above in the diagnosis phases (i.e., indicates that a wound in chronic inflammation will progress to acute inflammation, or an acutely inflamed wound will progress to proliferation). Remember a change in phase is a functional outcome prediction.

— Clean and stable open wound. Some wounds progress to proliferation but are not expected to close by secondary intention.

— Ready for surgical closure. This is the same as a clean and stable open wound; however, the plan is for surgical closure.

— Not expected to improve. In these cases of Medicare patients, nursing may remain with the patient if all other requirements are met BUT physical therapy is required to have a prognosis of excellent or good to continue treating the patient's wound.

Goals

Goals assist in determining the outcomes of care and therefore the effectiveness of care.

• Based on priorities that are dynamic and are stated as either short or long term.

— Short-term goals: small steps that move toward the long term goal and usually must be met before discharge or transfer to another level of care.

— Long-term goals: usually those that require continued attention by the client, family, and/or caregiver after discharge. May also be achieved if client is transitioned to custodial level of care in long term care from skilled level of care.

• Stated as broad guidelines that indicate overall direction of movement as a direct result of planned interventions.

Outcomes

Outcomes are the result of the interventions or activity that must be realistic, understandable, measurable, behavioral, achievable, specific, and individualized.

- Prevention and reduction:
  — Reduces, guards, or buffers against risks that generally exist either before or at the onset of a problem.
    ▪ A buffer attempts to diminish or reduce the risk with the intention of changing the progression of potential wounding, impairment, or disability.
  — The Braden Scale—or other risk assessment scale—may be used in the initial assessment and reassessment encounters to determine client risk and enable the practitioner to develop a plan to prevent wounding from developing.
- Controlled versus maintained (avoid the term *maintained* as this indicates lack of skilled care):
  — Maintained is not used as it implies no change; therefore, controlled is the better term as it indicates that an intervention has resulted in some (or total) stabilization of a specific condition such as edema that stabilizes from treatment to treatment.
  — One way to document this would be to state it as a functional outcome: "periwound edema controlled and wound demonstrates epithelialization" (this demonstrates the functional outcome as the wound healing even with edema remaining as it is controlled).
- Maximized:
  — Stated as a functional outcome it includes the intervention as well as result such as "performs ADLs in electric W/C pressure reduction cushion, has returned to work/leisure activities." This patient would usually be discharged from HHA not necessarily from SNF.
- Minimized:
  — Stated as a functional outcome it also includes the intervention and the result such as patient identified risk reduction method (state the method) to minimize wounding from shear and friction.
- AVOID: improved, provided, or promoted
  — Improved is too subjective; state the observed measurable changes in the wound.

— Provided is a practitioner's action, not an outcome.

— Promoted is a process, not an outcome.

• Behavioral terms to use in outcomes:

— Answer, apply, compare, choose, decrease, demonstrated, describe, explain, increase, participate, prepare, select, etc. AVOID learn, feel, understand, know, and accept.

CONSIDERATIONS IN ACUTE WOUNDS

• Primary intention:

— Stringent safeguards against infection

— Support client's immune system

— Some research indicates that wounds closed with the newer closure tapes develop increased resistance to infection more quickly and effectively than those sutured or stapled. Sutures and staples may allow bacteria under the skin.

  ▪ Tincture of benzoin placed on the skin and allowed to dry before application of the cloth strips creates longer wearing time for the strips. Remember that this tincture is destructive to fibroblasts and temporarily alters the pH of the skin to which it is applied. Using a skin barrier wipe such as 3M No Sting or Kendall Preppies may accomplish the same outcome without fibroblast destruction.

— If the wound is sutured or stapled keep it clean and dry until sutures or staples are removed.

— Dressing purpose is to support healing in a dry, low bacterial count (all skin has bacteria on it) environment.

  ▪ Remember: bacteria thrive in warm, dark, and moist environments so if dressings become moist and wet they should be changed (not reinforced) immediately.

• At the first encounter educate the client and caregiver that the purpose of the outpatient or home evaluations is to provide them support until one of them is able to perform the wound care.

*Indicates acute care or skilled nursing facility initial encounter or admission

— The practitioner develops a plan of care with the independence of the patient and caregiver as both a goal and an outcome.

- Consider referrals to OT, MSW*, PT*, WOC nurse, and RN to assist in this.
- Include in the first encounter:
  ○ Education on infection control*:
    - Dressings
    - Storage
    - Handwashing*
    - Keeping wound covered* (if part of POC)
    - Nutrition* (may have the client and caregiver keep a 72-hour diet and fluid log)
    - Disposal of used supplies*
- Homework*: activities the client and caregiver are to perform before the next encounter even if that encounter is later in the day. For example, on admission the client and caregiver are educated about handwashing for all care providers before wound evaluation or treatment. The client and caregiver are expected to observe and request when necessary for care providers to perform handwashing before wound evaluation or treatment is performed.

- Superficial:
- Stringent safeguards against infection
  — Keep wound covered to prevent shear, friction, and other trauma.
- Dressing purpose is to support healing in a dry, low bacterial count (all skin has bacteria on it) environment.
  — Remember: bacteria thrive in warm, dark, and moist environments so if dressings become wet they should be changed (not reinforced) immediately.

- Support client's immune system
- Continue evaluation for further, deeper tissue trauma
- Intervene with prevention techniques
- At the first encounter educate the client and caregiver that the purpose of the outpatient home encounters is to provide them support until one of them is able to perform the wound care.

  * Indicates acute care or skilled nursing facility initial assessment or admission

  — The practitioner develops a plan of care with the independence of the client and caregiver as both a goal and an outcome.

    ▪ Include in the first encounter:

      ○ Education on infection control*:

        • Dressings*
        • Storage
        • Handwashing*
        • Keeping wound covered* (if part of POC)
        • Nutrition* (may have the client and caregiver keep a 72-hour diet and fluid log if evaluation indicates client is at moderate to high risk of malnutrition)
        • Disposal of used supplies*

      ○ Educate regarding prevention techniques; include a practice or return demonstration*

      ○ Homework*: activities the client and caregiver are to perform before the next encounter even if that encounter is later in the day. For example, on admission the client and caregiver are educated about handwashing for all care providers before wound evaluation or treatment. The client and caregiver are expected to observe and request when necessary for care providers to perform handwashing before wound evaluation or treatment is performed.

- Delayed primary:
  — Stringent safeguards against infection

- Keep wound covered (moist healing is necessary)
- Dressing will require daily (at least) changes as IF the wound was contaminated with microorganisms or foreign bodies and this is the rationale for delayed closure. It may NOT require daily changes if this closure was chosen because there was a large tissue loss OR primary closure would have placed too much tension on the wound
- Dressing purpose is to support healing in a moist, low bacterial count (all skin had bacteria on it) environment.
- Remember: bacteria thrive in warm, dark, and moist environments so if dressings become wet they should be changed (not reinforced) immediately.

— Support client's immune system
— Continue evaluation for evidence of active infection either local or systemic
  - Intervene with infection prevention techniques
— Homework*: activities the client and caregiver are to perform before the next encounter even if that encounter is later in the day. For example, on admission the client and caregiver are educated about handwashing for all care providers before wound evaluation or treatment. The client and caregiver are expected to observe and request when necessary for care providers to perform handwashing before wound evaluation or treatment is performed.

• At the first encounter educate the patient and caregiver that the purpose of the outpatient or home encounters is to provide them support until one of them is able to perform the wound care.

   * Indicates acute care or skilled nursing facility initial assessment and admission

• The practitioner develops a POC with the independence of the client and caregiver as both a goal and an outcome.
   — Include in the first encounter:
     - Education on infection control*:

- Dressings*
- Storage
- Handwashing*
- Keeping wound covered* (if part of POC)
- Signs and symptoms of infection and to whom to report what and when.* May have patient and caregiver keep a log of temperatures and other vital signs; include CHHA in plan of vital signs measurement.
- Nutrition*: have client and caregiver keep a 72-hour diet and fluid log IF evaluation indicates patient is at moderate to high risk of malnutrition.
- Disposal of used supplies*
  - Educate regarding prevention techniques; include a practice or return demonstration*
  - Homework*: activities the client and caregiver are to perform before the next encounter even if that encounter is later in the day. For example, on admission the client and caregiver are educated about handwashing for all care providers before wound evaluation or treatment. The client and caregiver are expected to observe and request when necessary for care providers to perform handwashing before wound evaluation or treatment is performed.
- Subsequent encounters:
  - Evaluate client and caregiver adherence with homework*
  - Evaluate wound including measurements and description of periwound area*
  - Continue with education and homework at each encounter*
- Partial thickness:
  - Stringent safeguards against infection
    - Keep wound covered (moist healing is necessary)
    - Dressing requires daily changes ONLY if a dressing cannot contain at least 50% of the exudate in 24 hours

OR there is clinical evidence that the wound has been contaminated with microorganisms such as in a peri-anal stage II pressure ulcer. BEST is changing dressing less often; SNF challenge is reimbursement and skilled designation based on what the dressing consists of and the number of changes in 24 hours.

- Dressing purpose is to support healing in a moist, low bacterial count (all skin had bacteria on it) environment.
- Remember: bacteria thrive in warm, dark, and moist environments so if dressings become wet they should be changed (not reinforced) immediately.

— Support client's immune system

— Continue evaluation for evidence of active infection either local or systemic

- Intervene with infection prevention techniques

- At the first encounter educate the client and caregiver that the purpose of the outpatient or home encounters is to provide them support until one of them is able to perform the wound care.

* Indicates acute care or skilled nursing facility initial assessment and admission

— The practitioner develops a POC with the independence of the client and caregiver as both a goal and an outcome.

- Include in the first visit:
  ○ Education on infection control*:
    - Dressings*
    - Storage
    - Handwashing*
    - Keeping wound covered*
  ○ Signs and symptoms of infection and to whom to report what and when.* May have client and care giver keep a log of temperatures and other vital signs AND include CHHA in plan of vital signs measurement. In the acute care or skilled nursing setting

include the CNA in the plan of vital signs measurement including when to report immediately to the RN/LPN/LVN.

- ○ Nutrition*: have client and caregiver keep a 72-hour diet and fluid log IF evaluation indicates patient is at moderate to high risk of malnutrition
- ○ Disposal of used supplies*
- ○ Expectations of the dressing* such as hydrocolloids

- Educate* regarding all prevention techniques such as infection, shear, and friction; include a practice or return demonstration

- Homework*: activities the client and caregiver are to perform before the next encounter even if that encounter is later in the day. For example, on admission the client and caregiver are educated about handwashing for all care providers before wound evaluation or treatment. The client and caregiver is expected to observe and request when necessary for care providers to perform handwashing before wound evaluation or treatment is performed.

- Subsequent encounters:
  - — Evaluate client and caregiver adherence with homework*
  - — Evaluate wound including measurements and description of periwound area*
  - — Continue with education and homework at each visit*
- Secondary intention:
  - — Stringent safeguards against infection
    - Keep wound covered (moist healing is necessary)
    - Dressing will require daily (at least) changes as IF the wound was contaminated with microorganisms or foreign bodies and this is the rationale for delayed closure.
    - Dressing purpose is to support healing in a moist, low bacterial count (all skin had bacteria on it) environment.

- Remember: bacteria thrive in warm, dark, and moist environments so if dressings become wet they should be changed (not reinforced) immediately.
— Support client's immune system
— Continue evaluation for evidence of active infection either local or systemic
  - Intervene with infection prevention techniques
- At the first encounter educate the client and caregiver that the purpose of the outpatient or home encounters is to provide them support until one of them is able to perform the wound care.

* Indicates acute care or skilled nursing facility initial assessment and admission

— The practitioner develops a plan of care with the independence of the client and caregiver as both a goal and an outcome.
  - Include in the first encounter:
    o Education on infection control*:
      - Dressings*
      - Storage
      - Handwashing*
      - Keeping wound covered* (if part of POC)
      - Signs and symptoms of infection and to whom to report what and when.* May have client and caregiver keep a log of temperatures and/or other vital signs AND include CHHA in plan of vital signs measurement.
      - Nutrition*: have client and caregiver keep a 72-hour diet and fluid log.
      - Disposal of used supplies*
      - Educate* regarding all prevention techniques; include a practice or return demonstration
      - Homework*: activities the patient and caregiver are to perform before the next visit even if that visit is later in the day. For example, on admission the

client and caregiver are educated about handwashing for all care providers before wound evaluation or treatment. The client and caregiver are expected to observe and request when necessary for care providers to perform handwashing before wound evaluation or treatment is performed.

- Subsequent encounters:
  — Evaluate client and caregiver adherence with homework
  — Evaluate wound including measurements, description of periwound area, evidence of necrotic tissue, wound bioburden
  — Continue with education and homework at each encounter*

CHRONIC WOUND HEALING

Determination of amount of skin damage (Table 9–1).

- No reverse order staging once the ulcer is staged, it is always that stage. Be sure to indicate healing.
- Staging is NOT possible in the presence of slough, tissue necrosis, or eschar that hampers proper visualization of the wound bed and the wound should ONLY be thoroughly described by the health-care practitioner in these circumstances.

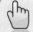

Nursing Alert
Staging of wounds is for use in pressure ulcers ONLY.

WOUND ASSESSMENT

The wound assessment is the written record, photograph, picture, drawing, and diagram of the progress of the wound and all the observations about that wound, data collection, and evaluation over time.

Table 9–1   Items to be Evaluated at Each Patient Encounter

STRUCTURES	PARTIAL/ FULL THICKNESS	DESCRIPTION AND EXAMPLES
Epidermis	**Partial**	Superficial, Stage I pressure ulcer, Grade 0 neuropathic foot, First degree burn
Epidermis and dermis	Partial	Abrasion, Stage II pressure ulcer, Grade 1 neuropathic foot, Skin graft donor site, Shave biopsy, Second degree burn
Subcutaneous Tissue	Full	Many lacerations and traumatic wounds, Stage III pressure ulcer, Grade 2 neuropathic foot, Third degree burn
Subcutaneous Tissue and Deep Fascia (bone)	Full	Some traumatic wounds, Stage IV pressure ulcer, Grade 3 neuropathic foot, Dehisced surgical wound, Third

When to assess or reassess any wound is determined by the level of care setting and the health-care providers in that setting as well as standards of practice and standards of care. It is important to remember that assessment and reassessment assist

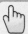

Nursing Alert
The cause (pathology) of any wound determines the treatment and drives the plan of care (POC). Therefore, before interventions can be initiated the type of wound and pathology must be known. The initial assessment of any client with skin, wounded or not, begins with a thorough history and physical examination.

the health-care providers in determining the success of the treatment and other interventions, achievable outcomes, and should guide decisions about product selection and change. Therefore reassessment of wounds should minimally be done:

- After the client returns from procedure or surgery
- Any time the dressing is changed
- Any time the wound deteriorates
- Any time there is a change in the odor from the wound
- Any time there is purulent exudate from the wound
- Any time there is any other significant change in the condition of the wound. Wounds should also be reassessed when there are significant changes in the general state of the health of the client that cannot be attributed to another cause.
- Any time the client has been sent to and returns from another care facility such as to an outpatient appointment
- According to the policy of the health-care organization

Components of wound assessment:[1]

- Anatomic location of wound
  — Use medical terminology (*left malleolus* rather than *left ankle*)
- Age of wound; the length of time client has had it; unless this is documented elsewhere in the medical record. Is it an acute or chronic wound?
- Drawing of human body; include wound location on this.
- Size
  — Actually measure the wound
  — State in centimeters (cm)
  — Length × width × depth
- Place the client on the surface of a clock. The health-care provider imagines this placement (Figure 9–1); it is not an actual placement.
- Shape
  — Oval, round, irregular, linear, other _____
- Stage I, II, III, IV (if a pressure ulcer)

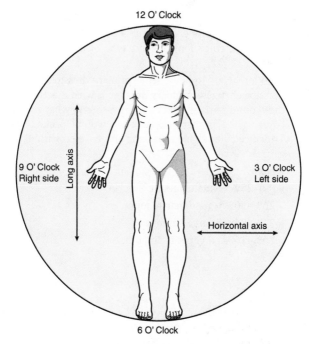

Figure 9–1 Wound Measurements. (Adapted with permission from Baranoski S, Ayello E. *Wound Care Essentials Practice Principles.* Philadelphia, PA: Lippincott Williams & Wilkins; 2004.)

- Sinus tract/tunneling
    — At ___ o'clock ___ cm.
- Undermining
    — From ___ o'clock to ___ o'clock ___ cm.
- Exudate
    — Color: serous (clear, watery plasma)
      Serosanguineous (plasma and red blood cells)
      Sanguineous (red blood cells)

— Consistency: thick, thin, or purulent (yellow, green, or brown; white blood cells and cellular debris and dead organisms; color may suggest type of infecting organism)

— Amount (refers to amount on primary dressing between dressing changes – primary dressing is what is actually on the wound surface; secondary dressing is what may be covering the primary dressing i.e. wound packed with 1-inch calcium alginate packing and covered with 4 × 4 gauze)

- None
- 0%–25% = small amount
- 26%–50% = moderate amount
- 51%–75% = large amount
- 76%–100% = copious amount

— Odor:

- None
- Mild
- Foul

— Surrounding (AKA periwound) skin:

- Intact/clear
- Macerated _____
- Erythematous _____
- Edematous _____
- Indurated _____
- Dry/flaky _____
- Other: _____

— Wound margins/edges:

- Attached (edges are attached to the sides of wound entire circumference)
- Not attached _____
- Edges rolled _____
- Sutures/staples intact

- Surgical incision approximated
- Surgical incision open _____
- Epithelialization present _____ cm
- Epithelialization not present

— Necrotic/devitalized tissue:
  - Not present
  - Present
  - Type
    - Yellow slough
    - Black
    - Soft
    - Hard
    - Stringy
    - Other
  - % of wound with necrotic/devitalized tissue
    - 100%
    - 75%
    - 50%
    - 25%
    - Other: ___%

— Wound/tissue bed:
  - Granulation tissue not present
  - Granulation tissue __%
  - Moist
  - Dry

— Neovascularization (blood vessels are visible/present):
  - Present
  - Not present

— Tenderness or pain:

— 0–10 scale (0 = no pain)
  - On touch
  - Anytime

- Only when performing wound care
- Other: _____ (specify)
— Pain management:
  - Not effective
  - Effective
— Wound status:
  - Improved: _____ date
  - Unchanged: _____ date
  - Healing: _____ date
  - Deteriorating: _____ date MD notified _____ date/time
  - Supportive therapy:
    ○ Compression
    ○ Pressure reduction mattress
    ○ Pressure reduction chair cushion
    ○ Amount of time up in chair with cushion
    ○ Off-loading
  - Patient's perception of quality of life _____
  - Referrals _____

WOUND CLEANSING CONCEPTS

Generic cleansing:
• Evaluate the wound and the dressing before initiating cleansing or other treatment. Remember to label the solution container with the date it was opened and first used.
  — If wound is essentially clean with little or no dressing residue or exudate, irrigate directly from the solution container with a catheter tip syringe or bulb syringe with water or normal saline is the most appropriate cleansing method. Use a gentle technique to diminish disruption of the healing process.
    ■ Best irrigation pressure to remove debris and bacteria from the wound is 5 to 15 psi. More pressure drives

bacteria into the tissues. A 19-gauge needle on 35 cc syringe delivers approximately 8 psi.

— If the wound demonstrates dressing residue, slough, necrotic tissue, dry or scaly skin, irrigate directly from the solution container with a catheter tip syringe or a bulb syringe with sterile water, normal saline, or a wound cleanser with a surfactant may assist in debris removal. Use a gentle technique and minimize direct contact with granulation tissue.

  ■ Best irrigation pressure to remove debris and bacteria from the wound is 5 to 15 psi. More pressure drives bacteria into the tissues. A 19-gauge needle on 35 cc syringe delivers approximately 8 psi.

— In both situations it is BEST to have the cleansing solution at room temperature. Cooler solutions reduce blood flow to the area.

— Protect the intact periwound skin from excessive moisture as it will macerate easily.

— In acute traumatic wounds or burns the use of a topical antiseptic in the early management will reduce the risk of infection from microorganisms and necrotic tissue. This technique reduces the level of bacteria in the wound and allows the immune system to destroy the rest.

— Rubbing, scrubbing, or other rough treatment of the wound and periwound tissue is to be avoided as this retards healing.

• Chronic wound cleansing:
  — Same principles apply as in generic cleansing
  — If debridement is necessary utilize appropriate techniques, NOT rubbing and scrubbing.
  — Refer to below for use of other cleansing solutions

• Infected wound cleansing:
  — Same principles apply as in generic cleansing
  — If debridement is necessary utilize appropriate techniques, NOT rubbing and scrubbing.
  — Refer to the details given in latter pages for use of other cleansing solutions

- Certain wound care solutions have the potential for wound healing impairment or prolonging healing time if caustic ones are selected and used inappropriately or for long term.
  — Antiseptic and antibacterial—all are cytotoxic

Treatment objectives of wound solution usage:

- Purpose is to gently remove debris without disruption of the healing process
- Use of antiseptic, antibacterial solutions should be for short time only and for specific, documented clinical reasons
- Wound care solutions for nonintact skin NOT skin care solutions and products
- Never scrub, rub, or disrupt the wound when cleansing or dressing
- ALWAYS protect healthy tissue from all cleansing solutions
- ALWAYS protect periwound tissue
- Cleansing or irrigating wounds
  — Use minimal force: pressure greater than 15 psi damages tissue and drives bacteria into the tissue
  — Whirlpool for necrotic tissue only
  — Pulsed lavage

Solutions used for wound care:

- Normal saline: physiologic, inexpensive, may be homemade, macerate wounded tissue or intact skin
- Acetic acid: glacial acetic acid in water, pH 2.9 to 3.3, exact action is not well understood but most microorganisms do not proliferate at low pH. It is an acid and all acids are bacteriostatic at low concentrations; bactericidal at higher concentrations. A 0.25% concentration is most often used in wound care and bladder irrigation.
  — May cause irritation and inflammation
  — Damages fibroblasts (more than it damages bacteria at these concentrations)
  — Discourages bacterial growth in surgical wounds and suppresses *Pseudomonas aeruginosa* growth in burns

- Burow/Domeboro solution (aluminum salts): usually found as 1% aluminum chlorhydrate, 10% aluminum acetate, 30% aluminum chloride hexahydrate, and 5% aluminum diacetate. These salts have strong antibacterial effects; completely inhibiting yeast's, gram positive, and gram negative bacteria in vitro. The in vivo recommended concentrations (1:20 or 1:40 of 5% aluminum diacetate) exert NO bacteriostatic or bactericidal effects. The solution has a mildly astringent effect.
  — External use only
  — May inhibit collagenase enzyme activity therefore cleanse wound thoroughly with normal saline before applying enzymes.
- Dakin's solution (Hypochlorites, Sodium hypochlorite, Chloramine-T): germicidal, deodorizing, and bleaching properties which most likely inhibit key enzymatic reactions within the microorganism. Protein denaturation and inactivation of nucleic acids.
  — NO concentration is harmless to cells including fibroblasts and endothelial cells; commonly used is 1/4 strength but may also be used at 1/8 strength
  — Chloramine-T retards development of collagen in healing skin defects and prolongs acute inflammatory phase
  — Sodium hypochlorite solutions dissolve blood clots, delay clotting, dry, and irritate the skin
  — For wound purposes usually 1/4 strength is ordered; however, in some unpublished research a solution of 1:40 has been shown to be effective
  — Protection of periwound and other intact skin is mandatory as is protection of clothing and the environment
- Hibiclens (chlorhexidine gluconate): 4% chlorhexidine gluconate and 4% isopropyl alcohol in a sudsing base. Contact bactericidal with antisepsis and persistent antimicrobial effects including gram positive and gram negative.
  — Works against yeast, molds, and viruses. In high temperatures it is sporicidal. Rapid acting with further reduction with repeated use.

— Safe to use on skin, for external use only; NOT for full-thickness wounds; avoid meninges contact

• Hydrogen peroxide: an oxidizing agent that releases molecular oxygen when in contact with tissues; this represents a very brief antimicrobial action.

— Toxic to fibroblasts unless diluted to more than 1:100

— Documented evidence that liberated oxygen has spread along fascial planes causing swelling and crepitation that has been misdiagnosed as invasion by gas-forming bacteria

— Documented evidence that use in wound cavities under pressure resulted in emboli

• Phisohex (hexachlorophene): a chlorinated phenolic compound that is an antibacterial cleanser

— Effective against gram positive bacteria, leaves residual on skin and is absorbed through skin which has a potential for toxicity to CNS

— Contraindicated in use on burned, denuded skin, or mucous membranes and in deep wounds

— When used as a cleanser, area must be cleansed for 3 minutes and rinsed thoroughly

• Povidone iodine solutions: polymer polyvinylpyrrolidone and iodine that is water soluble and slowly releases free iodine. Broad spectrum antimicrobial with unknown action. Activated in presence of blood and organic matter.

— Kills gram positive, gram negative, fungi, viruses, protozoa, and yeast. Destroys spores with moist contact of more than 15 minutes

— Clinical indications: prevention and treatment of surface infections such as degerm skin prior to invasive procedures

— 1:1000 dilution is the only one that has NO fibroblast toxicity (usual use is 10%)

— FDA has not approved antiseptic solution or surgical scrub solution for use in wounds

— Its ability to reach and kill bacteria in wounds is highly suspect due to the fact that the iodine must reach the bacterial cells in an active form and iodine is insoluble in water; tissue fluid is mostly water

— Long-term use may cause iodine toxicity

— Stains skin, clothing, and environment

- Soap and water: few studies but used in home care; probably not best for full thickness skin losses as a topical cleanser; soap does not get thoroughly rinsed out

  — Inexpensive and easily available. Evaluate bacterial count in water.

- Wound cleansers: various brands and components

  — Preservatives may cause burning

  — May be no more effective than normal saline

  — Some allergies have been reported to some components

Infected wounds:

- Identify and eliminate infections

  — Wound infection is 104 or 105 organisms per gram of tissue

    ▪ Wound infection definition: "the invasion and multiplication of microorganisms in wound tissue resulting in pathophysiologic effects or tissue injury."[2]

  — All chronic wounds are colonized (not the same as infection):

    ▪ Colonization refers to a state in which the wound surface has sustained colonization by microorganism replication without invasion of the tissue and no host immune response.[3]

  — Some colonizers are benefiting the host by preventing the adherence of more virulent microorganisms in the wound bed:

    ▪ Corynebacteria species

    ▪ Coagulase negative staphylococci

    ▪ Viridans stretococci

— Wound contamination refers to the presence of bacteria on the wound surface with no bacterial multiplication.

— Contamination and colonization are commonly found in wounds healing by secondary intention and are prerequisites for granulation formation.

— Wound infection prolongs inflammatory response, delays collagen synthesis, retards epithelialization, and increases tissue injury due to the bacterial competition for limited amounts of oxygen.

— Acute wounds are susceptible to skin flora invasion and the larger the loss of the surface area increases the susceptibility.

— Suspect a high bioburden of bacteria in a clean appearing wound that does not demonstrate healing or improvement within 14 days, if the wound is receiving the appropriate topical treatment.

— Chronic inflammation results in proliferation of fibroblasts and scar tissue.

— Infection may also affect the proliferative phase of wound healing by causing granulation tissue to become edematous, hemorrhagic, and fragile.

— Systemic infection signs:
  - Elevated body temperature
  - Elevated white cell count
  - Red streaks in the wound
  - Agitation or confusion in older adults who have not been agitated or confused, but also in those who have been but there is a change in the agitation or confusion
  - Elevated blood sugar in diabetics

— Local infection signs:
  - Skin erythema* or discoloration
  - Edema* in the wound and/or periwound area
  - Warmth* in the wound and/or periwound area
  - Induration in the wound and/or periwound area

- ▪ Increased pain* (may not always be in or around the wound)
- ▪ Purulent exudate (may/not have foul odor): known as signs of inflammation and can be related to tissue damage not caused by infection
- Surgical site infection (Table 9–2)
- Chronic wounds may demonstrate additional signs and symptoms of infection:
  - — Serous exudate with concurrent inflammation
  - — Delayed healing (lack of progress toward wound closure with no decrease in wound size may be the only sign in some wounds)
  - — Discoloration of granulation tissue
  - — Friable granulation tissue
  - — Pocketing at the base of the wound
  - — Foul odor
  - — Wound breakdown

NOTE: all chronic wounds are colonized. Have a specific clinical rationale for all wound cultures in the home or skilled nursing facility.

- Obtaining a wound culture:
  - — Cleanse wound with sterile normal saline or sterile water
  - — Remove wound debris
  - — Compress wound edges
  - — Culture with moistened (normal saline or culture media) swab and use 10 point method, broad Z-stroke, and firm pressure over entire wound bed—also known as Levine method

  OR

  - — Aspirate collection:
    - ▪ Palpate skin flaps and cellulitis areas
    - ▪ Prepare site
    - ▪ Sterile 3ml syringe or 22g needle

Table 9-2 CDC Criteria for Surgical Site Infection

The Centers for Disease Control and Prevention (CDC) has established the following criteria to define surgical site infection (SSI).

Superficial incisional SSI	Deep incisional SSI	Organ/space SSI

Involves only skin or subcutaneous tissue of the incision and at least one of the following:
• purulent drainage from the superficial incision
• organisms isolated from aseptically obtained culture of fluid tissue from the incision
• at least one of the following, unless negative culture:
  – pain or tenderness
  – localized swelling
  – redness or heat
  – incision opened by surgeon.
	Involves deep soft tissue (such as fascia and muscle layers) of the incision and at least one of the following:
	• purulent drainage from the deep incision but not organ/space
	• deep incision spontaneously opened by surgeon with one of the following symptoms, unless negative culture:
	  – fever greater than 100.4°F (38°C)
	  – localized pain
	  – an abscess
	• diagnosis of deep SSI by surgeon or attending physician.
		Involves any part of the anatomy (other than the incision) opened or manipulated during operation and at least one of the following:
		• purulent drainage from a drain placed in organ/space
		• organisms isolated from aseptically obtained culture of fluid or tissue in organ/space
		• an abscess or other evidence of infection
		• diagnosis of an organ/space SSI by a surgeon or attending physician.

- - Aspirate specimen
  - Transfer to culture medium
- Laboratory information
  - Date and time collected
  - Anatomical site and specific source
  - Type of specimen
  - Requested examination and tests
  - Diagnoses (primary/secondary)
  - Any therapy (topical, etc.)
- Do not culture eschar, slough, or devitalized tissue
- Specific treatment considerations for infected wounds:
  - Remove devitalized tissue (bacterial media)
  - Change dressings daily until infection resolved
  - Cleanse with appropriate solution such as a normal saline preparation: 1 quart water boiled for 5 minutes; add 2 teaspoons noniodized salt; allow to completely dissolve; covered in a tightly sealed glass or plastic container it can be stored, at room temperature, for 7 days.
  - Irrigation as the cleansing technique: minimize chemical and mechanical trauma to wound tissue; remove debris and contaminants
  - Refrain from using occlusive dressings and adhesives initially
  - Antiseptic agents
  - Topical antibiotics and treatments; limit therapy to 2 weeks
    - Silver 1% sulfadiazine (silvadene)
    - Double antibiotic ointment
    - Triple antibiotic ointment; more reactions to this than double due to presence of neomycin
    - Metronidazole 0.75%
  - Topical dressings impregnated with silver (selective use)
  - Systemic antibiotics

Infected wounds:

- Wound infection definition "the invasion and multiplication of microorganisms in wound tissue resulting in pathophysiologic effects or tissue injury."[2]
- Wound infection
  — Occurs in wound tissue NOT on the surface of the wound bed
  — Occurs in viable wound tissue NOT necrotic tissue, eschar, or other wound debris
  — Is caused by microbial invasion and multiplication in the wound
  — Is manifested by a host reaction or tissue injury
- Identify and eliminate infections
- Wound infection is 104 or 105 organisms per gram of tissue (AHRQ)[1]
  — β-hemolytic Streptococcus is a threat in wounds regardless of the number of organisms present
  — Wounds with ≥ 1,000,000 organisms per gram of tissue, milliliter of fluid, or swab is considered to be infected
  — Swab cultures 4+ are considered + for infection
- All chronic wounds are colonized (not the same as infection)
- Colonization refers to a state in which the wound surface has sustained colonization by microorganism replication without invasion of the tissue and no host immune response.[3]
- Some colonizers are benefiting the host by preventing the adherence of more virulent microorganisms in the wound bed:
  — Corynebacteria species
  — Coagulase negative staphylococci
  — Viridans streptococci
- Common organisms isolated from chronic wounds:
  — *Proteus mirabilis*
  — *Escherichia coli*
  — Streptococcus

— Staphylococcus

— *Psuedomonas*

— Corynbacteria

— *Bacteroides*

- Wound contamination refers to the presence of bacteria on the wound surface with no bacterial multiplication.

- Contamination and colonization are commonly found in wounds healing by secondary intention and are prerequisites for granulation formation.

- Wound infection prolongs inflammatory response, delays collagen synthesis, retards epithelialization, and increases tissue injury due to the bacterial competition for limited amounts of oxygen.

- Acute wounds are susceptible to skin flora invasion and the larger the loss of the surface area, the more increased the susceptibility.

- Suspect a high bioburden of bacteria in a clean appearing wound that does not demonstrate healing or improvement within 14 days if the wound is receiving the appropriate topical treatment.

- Chronic inflammation results in proliferation of fibroblasts and scar tissue.

- Infection may also affect the proliferative phase of wound healing by causing granulation tissue to become edematous, hemorrhagic and fragile.

- Fragile granulation tissue bleeds readily when gently manipulated with a sterile cotton-tipped applicator also known as a 6-inch applicator. This is often a symptom of wound infection.

- Discoloration of granulation tissue may also be a symptom of wound or ulcer infection and is represented by granulation tissue that is pale, dusky, or dull in color when compared to surrounding healthy tissue.

- Delayed healing equals no change, or an increase in the volume or surface area of the wound or ulcer over the preceding 4 weeks leads to delayed healing. Evaluate documentation for smaller wound dimensions or less wound depth 4 weeks before; suspect high bioburden, colonization, and possible infection.

- Pocketing at the base of a wound or ulcer represented by the presence of smooth, nongranulating pockets of ulcer tissue surrounded by beefy, red granulation tissue may also represent local infection.

- Small open areas of newly formed epithelial tissue that has not been caused by reinjury or trauma indicating wound breakdown are also representative of local infection.

- Systemic infection signs:
  — Elevated body temperature
  — Elevated white cell count
  — Red streaks in the wound

- Agitation or confusion in older adults who have not been agitated or confused but also in those who have been but there is a change in the agitation or confusion.

- Elevated blood sugar in diabetics
  — Blood sugars ≥ 200 prolongs healing in diabetics and non-diabetics when this is a consistent level.

- Local infection signs:
  — Skin erythema* or discoloration
  — Bright or dark red skin in a lighter colored person or darkening in a more darkly colored person that is immediately adjacent to the ulcer or wound opening is usually indicative of erythema

- Edema* in the wound and/or periwound area
  — Shiny, taut, or pitting in the skin adjacent to the ulcer or wound but "within 4 cm of the ulcer margin."[1] Determine this by measuring 4 cm away from the ulcer margin, pressing firmly with 1 or 2 fingers, releasing and waiting 5 seconds. Observe the indentation. The pitting should remain to be classified as pitting. Document exactly as it was determined.

- Warmth* and heat in the wound and/or periwound area
  - Increase in temperature of the skin adjacent to the ulcer or wound but within 4 cm of the ulcer margin that is detectable as compared to the skin 10 cm proximal to the wound. Using the posterior part of the hand or the anterior wrist, the appropriate area is felt for temperature variances. Document findings.

- Induration in the wound and/or periwound area is a hardening or firmness that is unusual in the specific area such as in the wound bed, at the wound margins, or in the ulcer/wound tissue around the wound margins. Document findings.

- Increased pain* that may not always be in or around the wound
  - If the patient reports increased pain in the wound or ulcer or the periwound is there since the wound or ulcer developed ask the patient to select from the following 4 statements:
    1. I can't detect pain in ulcer area.
    2. I have less ulcer pain now than I had in the past.
    3. The intensity of the ulcer pain has remained the same since the ulcer developed.
    4. I have more pain now than I had in the past.

  If the patient selects number 4, his or her pain is increasing. Write N/A if the patient cannot respond to the question.[1]

- Purulent exudate (may/not have foul odor)
  - Tan, creamy, yellow, or green thick fluid that is present on a dry gauze dressing removed from the wound or ulcer 1 hour after the wound or ulcer was appropriately cleaned and dressed of purulent exudate.[1]

  *Known as signs of inflammation and can be related to tissue damage not caused by infection.

- Surgical Site Infection (see Table 9–2)
- Chronic wounds may demonstrate additional signs and symptoms of infection:
  - Serous exudate with concurrent inflammation

— Delayed healing is a lack of progress toward wound closure with no decrease in wound size may be the only sign in some wounds
— Discoloration of granulation tissue
— Friable granulation tissue
— Pocketing at the base of the wound
— Foul odor
— Wound breakdown

NOTE: all chronic wounds are colonized. Have a specific clinical rationale for all wound cultures in the home or skilled nursing facility.

- Obtaining (before administering antibiotics) a wound culture (use sterile technique):
  — Cleanse wound with sterile normal saline or sterile water
  — Remove wound debris
  — Compress wound edges
  — Culture with moistened normal saline or culture media swab (use 10 point method, broad Z-stroke); obtain enough specimen
  — Use firm pressure over entire wound bed—also known as Levine method—is now thought to be more effective if swab method is only choice for wound culture available.
  OR
  — Aspirate collection
  — Palpate skin flaps and cellulitis areas
  — Prepare site
  — Sterile 3ml syringe and 22-gauge needle
  — Aspirate specimen
  — Transfer to culture medium
- Laboratory information:
  — Date and time collected
  — Anatomical site and specific source
  — Type of specimen

— Requested examination and tests
— Diagnoses (primary/secondary)
— Any therapy (topical, etc.)

- Transport to laboratory quickly in appropriate container with appropriate conditions.
- Do not culture eschar, slough or devitalized tissue.
- Specific treatment considerations for infected wounds:

  — Remove devitalized tissue (bacterial media)
  — Change dressings daily until infection resolved
  — Cleanse with appropriate solution of normal saline preparation: 1 quart water boiled for 5 minutes; add 2 teaspoons noniodized salt; allow to completely dissolve; covered in a tightly sealed glass or plastic container it can be stored at room temperature for 7 days.
  — Irrigation as the cleansing technique: minimize chemical and mechanical trauma to wound tissue; but remove debris and contaminants
  — Refrain from using occlusive dressings and adhesives (initially)
  — Antiseptic agents
  — Topical antibiotics and treatments, limit therapy to 2 weeks
  — Silver 1% sulfadiazine (silvadene)
  — Double antibiotic ointment
  — Triple antibiotic ointment (more reactions to this than double due to present of neomycin)
  — Metronidazole 0.75%
  — Topical dressings impregnated with silver (selective use)
  — Systemic antibiotics

MOIST WOUND HEALING

The hypothesis comes from the pathophysiology of skin. If one of the functions of the intact epidermis is to retain the moisture of the cells that lie beneath it then it would seem that healing of any injury to the tissues below the epidermis would require a maintenance of that same moisture. Therefore, the concept of "moist wound healing" exists although it has taken nearly 2000 years for humankind to understand this seemingly simple concept.

Partial thickness wounds:

- If covered with moisture-retentive dressings, they epithelialize two times faster than identical wounds left open to air *in pigs*.[4]

- Epithelial cells can migrate in a moist environment on the wound bed surface to close a partial thickness wound = reepithelialization = no scar formation.

- Epithelial cells can burrow underneath the wound bed in a dry wound but the healing time is longer with more chance of unplanned events occurring as in local infection.

Objective of moist wound healing:

- Create an environment as close to the body's own "healing environment" as possible.

  — The body's healing environment is similar to an intact blister; therefore, the best wound healing treatment will create a humid (not wet) environment that:

    ▪ Promotes rapid healing
    ▪ Acts as a protective barrier
    ▪ Decreases or eliminates pain
    ▪ Requires few/or no changes
    ▪ Can be cost effective if used appropriately
    ▪ Provides autolytic debridement

Management of Necrotic Tissue

- Definition of terms

  — Slough: is generally moist yellow or tan with a thin, mucous, or stringy quality (devitalized connective tissue).

  — Eschar: is generally brown or black and may be both dry and leathery, hard, or soft and spongy (dehydrated).

Necrotic tissue is dying or dead tissue. It changes in color, adherence to wound bed and edges, and consistency as the preceding tissue dies. The amount and the color can gauge the severity of necrotic tissue. Initially this dying tissue is white or gray becoming yellow or tan and finally it becomes brown or black. As this tissue continues to dry out or desiccate the consistency changes. At the initial stages the tissue is often hydrated and therefore mucoid in consistency becoming stringy with more lumps as the tissue continues to die. The final stage of death is represented by hard, dry, leathery tissue. The level of tissue death is important in determining the treatment of the wound as well as determining prevention strategies. When differing levels of tissue die they present differently:

- The presentation of necrotic or devitalized tissue:
  — Subcutaneous tissue form yellow, stringy slough.
  — Muscle tissue may form a similar type to subcutaneous but the dead tissue is generally thicker and more tenacious.
  — According to histological research, hard, black eschar is skin death with full thickness loss.
  — If the wound has suffered prolonged ischemia the dying tissues are often grey and the surrounding skin may take on a bluish hue or become white due to devitalization. This necrotic tissue may be firmly adherent, thick, desiccated, and black or grey in color.
  — The water content of the tissue and the depth of damage determine the tenacity of adherence of the tissue debris to the wound bed:
    - More water content = less adherence
    - Less water content = more adherence
    - The more necrotic tissue, the more adherent
  — Expected outcomes: if eschar becomes nonadherent to the wound, the longer the healing time. The necrotic tissue acts as a bacterial medium as well as a physical barrier to epidermal resurfacing, contraction, and granulation.

— In the early phase of pressure ulcers, the tissue may change color and be indurated with either purple or black discoloration of the intact skin.

— Neuropathic or neurotrophic wounds most often present with hyperkeratosis in the periwound area rather than tissue necrosis. In appearance this often looks like callous formation.

— Venous wounds will often present with yellow fibrinous slough in the wound bed or covering the wound but they may also develop eschar.

Wound Debridement

- Obstructs epithelial migration
- Promotes bacterial growth
- Interferes with "normal" granulation
- Inhibits wound contraction
- Promotes occlusion
- May increase amount of nursing time as it often creates a situation that requires more dressing or linen changes
- Often has foul odor
- Objectives of debridement:
  — Promote and develop healthy wound bed that supports tissue regeneration
  — Reduce bioburden of wound; prevent and control infection in deteriorating wounds.
  — Remove necrotic, devitalized tissue without causing harm to surrounding tissue or the host or organization
    ▪ Selective
    ▪ Nonselective
    ▪ Zero to minimal blood loss
    ▪ Cost and time efficient
    ▪ Technical ease and availability
- General indications for wound debridement:

— Devitalized or necrotic tissue present in otherwise viable wound
— Advancing cellulitis
— Sepsis
— Abscess
• General contraindications for wound debridement:
— Clean, granulating, stable wounds
— Noninfected, ischemic wounds with poor perfusion
— Inappropriate for overall treatment goals
— Heel ulcers with dry, stable, nonsymptomatic eschar (NPUAP, AHCPR, 1994) (AHCPR now known as AHRQ)
— No edema, erythema, fluctuance (fluid wave), or drainage. The eschar is acting as a barrier to infection. Focus on preventing trauma to foot.
• Debridement as a wound management tool:
— Autolytic debridement: breakdown of necrotic tissue by body's own leukocytes. Requires a moisture retentive dressing, which rehydrates the dead tissue thereby facilitating leukocyte and enzyme action and movement (Tables 9–3 and 9–4).
— Choices of method and dressing are dependent on wound type such as arterial ischemic ulcer, pressure ulcer, and venous stasis ulcer.

Autolytic debridement product selection:
• Black or brown HARD eschar
— Transparent film dressing is best for pressure ulcers not with venous disease ulcers or arterial ischemic ulcers
— Hydrocolloid is best for venous disease ulcers; appropriate with pressure ulcers or arterial ischemic ulcers
— Hydrogel is best for venous disease ulcers; appropriate with pressure ulcers; best with arterial ischemic ulcers
— Expected outcomes:
  ▪ Eschar nonadherent to wound edges

Table 9–3   Indications and Contraindications of Autolytic
Debridement

Indications	Contraindications
Most beneficial on dry eschar. Patient with normal, intact inflammatory response. Partial/full thickness wounds with adherent necrotic tissue. Patient unable to tolerate other debridement methods or other debridement methods are not available.	Not for use on dry gangrene or dry ischemia unless a vascular consult has verified the circulatory status and approved of this debridement as in pressures on heels, arterial ulcers, some diabetic foot wounds, infection, cellulitis, suspected abscess, deep tissue destruction, or advancing cellulitis.
All necrotic wounds if blood flow has not been compromised	
May require cross (X) hatching	

- Lifting of necrotic tissue from wound edges
- Softening of necrotic tissue
- Necrotic tissue color change to yellow or tan
- Black or brown soft and soggy eschar or yellow or tan slough (soft and stringy, fibrinous, or mucoid)
  — Hydrocolloid is best for pressure ulcers and venous disease ulcers but not arterial ulcers
  — Hydrogel is best for venous disease ulcers, appropriate with pressure ulcers, best with arterial ischemic ulcers
  — Expected outcomes:
    - Lifting of necrotic tissue from wound bed
    - Change in consistency of necrotic tissue to stringy or mucoid
    - Change in tissue color to yellow or white
    - Change in amount of necrotic tissue covering the wound; usually a gradual decrease until majority of wound is clean

Table 9–4   Advantages and Disadvantages of Autolytic Debridement

Advantages	Disadvantages***
Quick: initial debridement in 4 to 6 days, overall 14 days. Readily available in most care settings. Noninvasive, painless. Facilitates sharp debridement through softening and hydrating necrotic tissue. Pain-free if adequate tissue perfusion.	Patient and caregiver education regarding appearance of autolyzing wound, color, odor, exudate, and need for dressing to remain in place. Monitor for infection. May need to score eschar and remove loose tissue first.
Selective.	Increased potential for periwound maceration.
Low cost.	May cause periwound skin tearing if removed improperly.
Effective with slough, fibrin, and eschar.	Slower than sharp methods. Useful in conjunction with mechanical or sharp methods.

- Consider using hydrocolloid strips or skin barrier wipe to create "window" around dressing if patient's skin is sensitive to adhesive or maceration is a concern before next dressing change and evaluation.
  — Educate patient and family concerning accumulation of fluid under dressing as a normal part of the debridement process and the distinctive odor of hydrocolloid.

*** Remember transparent film dressings have a tendency to lift off prematurely in the presence of large amounts of exudate. Hydrocolloids leak emitting a distinctive odor that may be troubling to some family members and patients.

Chemical Debridement

- Tables 9–5 and 9–6 list advantages/disadvantages
- Enzymatic Debridement: using enzymatic solutions or ointments

Table 9–5 Indications and Contraindications of Chemical Debridement

Indications	Contraindications
All necrosis; best with moist wounds. Substrate drugs act upon fibrous proteins which must be present in wound i.e. collagen, fibrin, protein, etc. When occlusive dressings are not appropriate.	Sensitivity to components. Drug specificity. Suspected abscess, deep tissue destruction, or advancing cellulitis.
Dry eschar X hatch method	Not for use in clean wounds
Match the enzyme type with the tissue type. Patient not a candidate for sharp or surgical debridement. As an adjunct to sharp or surgical debridement.	Not for use on dry gangrene or dry ischemia unless a vascular consult has verified the circulatory status and approved of this debridement as in pressures on heels, arterial ulcers, and some diabetic foot wounds. Not for use with wounds with poor perfusion.

to remove necrotic tissue. Note: it is best to use a normal saline moist gauze covering (if the particular enzyme requires a moist dressing) and normal saline wound cleansing as some of the enzymes are inactivated by metals–lead, mercury or silver–that may be found in other solutions.

Black or brown eschar or yellow or tan slough:

• May be used on pressure ulcers, venous disease ulcers, arterial ischemic ulcers. Not for use on neurologic, neurotrophic ulcers. Panafil® debriding, healing ointment, a Healthpoint product, may be used to lift necrotic tissue from wound edges, soften necrotic tissue, change necrotic tissue color, and change eschar to slough.

• Enzyme Types:

• Granulex: Trypsin and balsum of Peru

— Mildly proteolytic

Table 9–6 Advantages and Disadvantages of Chemical Debridement

Advantages	Disadvantages
Tissue selectivity. Most are widely available in all care settings.	Stop when wound is clean. May cause transient pain, burning, bleeding, or periwound dermatitis.
Effective in conjunction with other debridement techniques.	May be slow; 14 to 30 days. May be labor intensive. Eschar requires adequate scoring for enzyme penetration.
Some are cost effective. May provide odor control.	Some require moist cover dressings and some are costly.
May be used with compatible antimicrobial.	Some require treatment every 8 hours. May require refrigeration.
	Nurse practitioner or physician order is required.
Facilitates sharp debridement through softening or loosening of necrotic tissue.	Manufacturer's guidelines must be followed. May require a specific pH range for effectiveness.
	Monitor for infection and burning with treatment.

- Santyl: Collagenase
  — Digests collagen
  — Digests denatured protein
- Panafil with chlorophyll (stains tissue deep green and color may be confused with infection)
  — Papain, urea, chlorophyllin, and copper
  — Proteolytic
  — Mild deodorant
- Accuzyme
  — Papain and urea
  — Proteolytic

Table 9–7 Indications and Contraindications of Maggot
Therapy

Indications	Contraindications
Sharp debridement may cause major damage to surrounding tissues.	Wounds with or near exposed or damaged blood vessels or nerves.
Failure of traditional methods especially for severe infections. Protect periwound area.	

- Expected Outcomes:
  — Generally, softening and removal of majority or all of devitalized tissue. In some cases, softening and pulling away from edges of devitalized tissue to prepare for sharp debridement may be the goal.
- Apply one-eighth inch of enzyme to the wound or ulcer after ascertaining that the appropriate selection has been made and the product does not harm granulation tissue.
  — Protect intact skin from contact with enzyme as maceration may occur.
  — Cover wound or ulcer with appropriate dressing and change according to manufacturer's or FDA's recommendations.
- Patient education
  — Some transient tingling or stinging pain may be felt from the enzymatic action when it is first applied but other increases in pain are not to be expected and should be reported to the health-care provider.
  — Educate patient and caregiver about signs and symptoms of infection and to whom to report.
  — Document education and patient and caregiver response.
- Remember some products require refrigeration.

Table 9–8 Advantages and Disadvantages of Maggot Therapy

Advantages	Disadvantages
Rapid debriding (200 to 600 larvae consume 10 to 15 grams of necrotic tissue per day).	Availability of larvae. Lack of acceptance from patient, staff, providers, and surveyors.
Infrequent dressing changes.	
Infection prevention and control. Odor control.	Crawling sensation if not confined to wound surface.
Inexpensive.	May damage surrounding epidermis.
Selective.	Skin barrier required to cover intact periwound skin to eliminate pruritus. Dressings must confine larvae to wound.

- Maggots: secrete proteolytic and antibacterial agents which liquefy necrotic tissue absorbed by the larvae. These secretions seem to stimulate granulation tissue (Tables 9–7 and 9–8).
- Expected outcomes:
  — Removal of all or majority of devitalized tissue in relatively short time
- Patient education:
  — Dressings should be removed by health-care professional if at all possible.
  — Some patients report a tickling sensation from the movement of the larva in the wound.
  — Can increase wound pain, particularly in ischemic leg ulcers.
  — Document education and patient and caregiver response.
- Remember: care should be taken to avoid bursting maggots since some patients can have anaphylactic reactions to larval protein.

Table 9–9   Indications and Contraindications of Sodium
             Hypochlorite

Indications	Contraindications
Malodorous wounds when infection is a risk and sharp debridement is not appropriate. DC when risks to tissue outweigh benefits due to fibroblast cytotoxicity.	Toxic to granulation tissue, granulation and epithelialization processes. Must protect periwound skin with skin barrier to eliminate damage.

Sodium Hypochlorite (Dakin 0.25% to 0.5%): action separates and digests necrotic dermis, fascia, and blood clots (Tables 9–9 and 9–10).

Expected outcomes:

- Removal of all or majority of devitalized tissue in relatively short time
- Separation of devitalized tissue from intact tissue
- Decrease in healing while using the solution
- Rapid decrease in odors
- Drying of periwound and ulcer tissue if not protected
- May increase pain on application

Table 9–10   Advantages and Disadvantages of Sodium
              Hypochlorite

Advantages	Disadvantages
Readily available in most care settings. Inexpensive.	Nonselective.
Odor control.	"Bleach" odor.
Antimicrobial, antiviral, antifungal.	0.5% is preferred for debridement but may be too strong for many patients; this strength solution may be more difficult to obtain.

Table 9–11   Indications and Contraindications of Mechanical Debridement

Indications	Contraindications
Contaminated wounds with necrotic or devitalized tissue.	Hard, dry eschar covering the wound.
	Clean, non-exudating, granulating wounds.

Patient education

- Specific to patient situation
- Document education and patient and caregiver response.

Mechanical Debridement

Mechanical debridement (Tables 9–11 and 9–12) is a mechanical means or outside force used to remove necrotic tissue and generally includes:

- Wound irrigation
  - Syringe (catheter tip not bulb syringe) or 35 cc syringe with 19g plastic catheter tip that equals 8 psi pressure
  - Pulsatile high pressure lavage (pulsed lavage)

Table 9–12   Advantages and Disadvantages of Mechanical Debridement

Advantages	Disadvantages
Inexpensive if using 35-cc syringe with 19-gauge catheter and Normal Saline. Irrigating tip must be within 1 to 2 inches of the wound surface.	Time and labor intensive. Protective equipment must be worn to protect from splash.
Readily available.	
Decreases bacterial burden economically and simply.	May cause periwound maceration if care is not exercised.

Table 9–13 Indications and Contraindications of Pulsative High-pressure Lavage

Indications	Contraindications
Heavily contaminated, large soft tissue wounds with tunneling and/or undermining.	Any wound where the force could damage critical anatomy (i.e., major vessel, cavity linings, exposed nerves, tendon, bone, grafts, flaps).
Whirlpool is not available or appropriate (e.g., obesity, critically ill, contractures, etc).	Clean, nonexudating, granulating wounds.
	Patients on anticoagulants or who are insensate.
	Pain not manageable with procedure.

  — Continuous high pressure irrigation (OR)
  — Wet to dry dressings (gauze dressing with various solutions)
  — Whirlpool
  — Osmotic pressure
- Mechanical debridement
- Irrigation: use of physical force on the wound surface to soften, loosen, or remove necrotic or devitalized tissue as well as wound debris and bacteria. Used in conjunction with other debridement methods.
- Continuous high pressure fluid is delivered at 4 to15 psi to the wound surface.
- Pulsative (pulsatile) high pressure lavage: fluid delivered at 0 to 60 psi to wound surface by a pulsing delivery system that is combined with suction. The pulsative effect is to loosen debris, devitalized, or necrotic tissue. Large volumes of solution (water or normal saline) flush the wound (Tables 9–13 and 9–14).
- Whirlpool: water immersion and agitation of an extremity or the entire body. This debridement method is thought to

Table 9–14 Advantages and Disadvantages of Pulsative High-pressure Lavage

Advantages	Disadvantages
Possible to perform procedure at the bedside.	Not available in all care settings.
Could replace whirlpool: less infection risk and may be less costly.	Requires training and skill.
Facilitates sharp debridement due to loosening and softening action.	Cost and reimbursement. Labor and time intensive.
Length of time for debridement usually 14 days but dependent on tissue type and amount to be debrided.	Must utilize personal protective equipment to protect from splash.
	No controlled studies supporting claims of rapid granulation and epithelialization available.

Table 9–15 Indications and Contraindications of Whirlpool Therapy

Indications	Contraindications
Large surface wounds with copious, thick exudate, slough, or adherent necrotic tissue.	Immune-suppressed patients or those with suspected low resistance to infection or with renal or cardio pulmonary failure.
	Deep tunneling wounds or clean, granulating wounds.
	Depressed CNS function.
	Dry gangrene or tissue with poor perfusion.
	Phlebitis or lower extremity venous compromise or edema.
	Neuropathic extremity.

Table 9–16   Advantages and Disadvantages of Whirlpool Therapy

Facilitates sharp debridement due to softening, loosening, and hydrating necrotic tissue.	Wound at risk of water born infection unless scrupulous attention to infection control. Discontinue when debridement achieved. Jets of the whirlpool should not be close to or directed on to the wound.
Controls odor. Selective.	Superhydration or maceration of skin and wound with an alteration in the skin pH.
Warmth may enhance cellular activity and perfusion while in the whirlpool.	Not available in all care settings and may be costly.
Length of time for debridement dependent on amount and type of devitalized or necrotic tissue, usually 2 to 4 weeks.	Labor and time intensive. Water temperature must be selected based on patient's condition and etiology of the wound.
	Vigorous rinsing after each use of the whirlpool is necessary to reduce bacterial counts. Pseudomonas aeruginosa is common. Patients and health-care workers subjected to aerosolization.
	Patient may experience pain from the whirlpool itself or simply the action of being taken to the whirlpool.

loosen, soften, and remove necrotic or devitalized tissue and wound debris. There are some who subscribe to the hypothesis that it also enhances local tissue perfusion (however, no evidence of this has been published) (Tables 9–15 and 9–16).

Suggested orders

• 10 to 20 minutes QD to BID, water temperature 80° to 92°F (26°–33°C) for tepid or 92° to 96°F (33.3°–35.5°C) for neutral.

Table 9–17 Indications and Contraindications of Osmotic Debridement

Indications	Contraindications
Full thickness wounds with moderate to large amounts of exudate and devitalized or necrotic tissue.	Hard, dry eschar. Partial thickness wounds. Wounds with minimal exudate.
Patient with normal inflammatory response.	

Expected outcomes:

- Removal of all or majority of devitalized tissue in relatively short time and may be used in conjunction with enzymatic debridement.

- Separation of devitalized tissue from intact tissue to prepare for sharp debridement.

- Patient education

  — Do not place wound near jets in whirlpool

  — Take or request pain medication before treatment as necessary

  — Specific to patient situation

  — Document education and patient and caregiver response.

  — Length of time patient is able to tolerate treatment

  — Special tub solutions as ordered, temperature, etc.

- Osmotic: Agents absorb or hold in suspension exudate, wound debris, and bacteria. This is used in conjunction with other debridement methods such as sharp and supports autolysis (Tables 9–17 and 9–18).

- Wet to Dry/Gauze Dressings: direct, blunt force to remove devitalized or necrotic tissue. This is considered outdated treatment for granulating wounds and may not be the most appropriate debridement technique for other wounds (Tables 9–19 and 9–20).

Table 9–18 Advantages and Disadvantages of Osmotic Debridement

Advantages	Disadvantages
Available in many forms (e.g., beads, ropes, granules, gels, pastes, and nonwoven fibrous mats).	May be difficult to apply depending on location and configuration of wound and product formulation.
Facilitates sharp debridement as it supports autolysis.	Not available in all care settings.
Less costly than some other debridement methods.	Requires a secondary dressing and securement.
Eliminates dead space.	Must monitor for infection. Discontinue when debridement completed.
Selective.	Length of time to debridement dependent on tissue type and amount; usually 3 weeks or less.

NOTE: if the order is for a wet to dry dressing, it means the dressing is intended to dry out before being removed.

- Gauze and normal saline: if the gauze dressing has been in contact with wounded tissue, according to research by Kim et al the dressing acts as an osmotic dressing.[1,5]
  - — Water evaporates and the saline becomes hypertonic
  - — The body wants to maintain homeostasis by reestablishing isotonicity, therefore wound fluid is drawn into the dressing
    - Wound fluid contains
      - ○ Water
      - ○ Proteins
      - ○ Blood
    - The wound fluid forms an impermeable layer on the dressing preventing wound fluid from "wetting" the gauze and the dressing dries out.

Table 9–19   Indications and Contraindications of Wet-to-Dry and Gauze Dressings

Indications	Contraindications
Moist wounds with small amounts of devitalized or necrotic tissue.	Never on granulation or reepithelializing tissue.
Infected wounds.	Painful when removed; usually requires premedication. The dressing is not intended to be moistened before removal and doing so is contradictory to the order.
Wounds with tunnels or sinus tracts.	
Most beneficial on soft slough but may be used on hard eschar (longer time for results).	Not for use on dry gangrene or dry ischemia unless a vascular consult has verified the circulatory status and approved of this debridement such as in pressure on heels, arterial ulcers, some diabetic foot wounds.

Table 9–20   Advantages and Disadvantages of Wet-to-Dry and Gauze Dressings

Advantages	Disadvantages
Inexpensive and readily available in all care settings.	Rarely applied or removed correctly.
Nonselective.	Removal may cause bleeding and pain. This interrupts wound healing if emerging granulation tissue is affected.
	Time and labor intensive. Supply use may be more costly.
	Length of time for debridement difficult to predict.

Table 9–21   Indications and Contraindications of Surgical
              Debridement

Indications	Contraindications
Full thickness wounds with presence of abscess, deep tissue destruction, or sepsis and large amounts of devitalized or necrotic tissue.	Patient not a candidate for surgery. Major coagulopathy.
Preparation of wound for flap or graft.	

- This "dried out" dressing is then removed from the wound and wherever it adheres to wound tissue, it may cause reinjury of the wound.
  - Reinjury results in pain and delayed healing according to Ovington.[6]
— Additionally, during the drying of the gauze dressing, the local tissue cools as water is evaporating. Studies have shown that reduced tissue temperatures have been found in these gauze covered wounds of 77° to 80.6°F (25°–27°C). Reduced wound temperature results in:
  - Local vasoconstriction
  - Hypoxia
  - Impaired leukocyte mobility
  - Impaired phagocytic efficiency
  - Increased affinity of hemoglobin for O_2
All of which result in impaired wound healing.[6]
- Expected outcomes:
  — Debridement partial or complete
- Patient education
  — Specific to patient situation
  — Document amount of gauze and solution used at each treatment and storage of supplies.

Table 9–22 Advantages and Disadvantages of Surgical Debridement

Advantages	Disadvantages
Fast and efficient. Length of time to debridement is length of procedure time.	Need OR conditions, highly invasive, anesthesia required, labor, time intensive. Surgeon must perform. Costly.
	Transient bacteremia.
	Pain.

— Document education, patient tolerance of treatment, and patient and caregiver response to education.

- Surgical debridement: sterile excision of devitalized, necrotic, and vascular tissue (wide excision). Generally done to prepare patient for surgical closure of wound. Physician required to perform this in the long-term care setting (Tables 9–21 and 9–22).

Expected outcomes:

- Rapid, one-time or staged procedure to remove all/majority of devitalized tissue or to remove callous to healthy, perfused tissue.

Table 9–23 Indications and Contraindications to Laser Therapy

Indications	Contraindications
Full thickness wounds with large amounts of devitalized or necrotic tissue.	
Debilitated patients unable to tolerate general anesthetic, long, conservative course of debridement, blood loss, or infection potential.	
Preparation of wound for grafting.	

Table 9-24 Advantages and Disadvantages of Laser Therapy

Advantages	Disadvantages
Fast, efficient. Allows surgical access to body cavities and inaccessible areas. General anesthesia not usually necessary.	Requires skill, surgeon must perform. May require regional anesthetic and/or hospitalization.
Renders wound bed aseptic. Bloodless field.	
Debridement is immediate.	

Patient education
- Specific to patient situation
- Document education, patient tolerance of treatment, and patient and caregiver response to education.
- Laser (CO_2): vaporization of necrotic tissue when light waves heat water in the tissues (Tables 9–23 and 9–24).

Expected outcomes:
- Rapid, one-time or staged procedure to remove all or majority of devitalized tissue or to remove callous to healthy, perfused tissue.

Patient education
- Specific to patient situation
- Document education, patient tolerance of treatment, and patient and caregiver response to education.
- Sharp or conservative sharp debridement: removal of loose, avascular tissue without pain or bleeding, using sterile instruments. Performed by physician, physician assistant, and registered nurse practitioner. Physical therapist and registered nurse can perform if follow special training and written policy, procedure, and protocol developed by agency (Tables 9–25 and 9–26).
- Black or brown eschar, or yellow or tan slough all types:

Table 9–25 Indications and Contraindications to Sharp or Conservative Sharp Debridement

Indications	Contraindications
Gross tissue necrosis. Partial or full thickness wounds with loose, avascular tissue.	**NOT** for use on **dry gangrene** or **dry** ischemia unless a vascular consult has verified the circulatory status and approved of this debridement as in pressure on heels, arterial ulcers, and some diabetic foot wounds. Noninfected, ischemic wound with dry eschar and poor perfusion.
	Patients at increased risk of bleeding or with impaired clotting.
	Heel ulcers with dry eschar and without edema, erythema, fluctuance, or exudate.
	Patient cannot remain stationary for length of time to perform procedure.
	Densely adherent necrosis.
	Not possible in all settings.

— May be used on pressure ulcers, venous disease ulcers, arterial ischemic ulcers, and neuropathic or neurotrophic ulcers (saucerization or callous removal) either one time or sequentially.

— Expected outcomes:

  ■ Removal or elimination of all or part of necrotic tissue dependent on multiple variables

  ■ Chronic inflammation halting due to removal of necrotic tissue and wound debris

  ■ Restarting of healing edges

  ■ Drainage of abscess

Table 9–26   Advantages and Disadvantages of Sharp or
Conservative Sharp Debridement

Advantages	Disadvantages
Fast, efficient if provider is skilled. May take only one time.	May be sequential.
Used in conjunction with other debridement treatments.	Requires expertise and skill.
May be cost effective.	Possible non-reimbursement for non-physician.
Performed at bed side. Available in most care settings.	Requires skill to perform accurately and efficiently.
Topical anesthetic not usually necessary.	Possible transient bacteremia.
Selective.	
Rapid effect.	Length of time to debridement dependent on type and amount of necrotic avascular tissue, usually immediate to within 7 days.
May cause chronic wound to become an acute wound.	Only minor bleeding, if any should occur (control with pressure and/or $AgNO_3$ sticks).

• Patient education
   — Specific to patient situation
   — Document education, patient tolerance of treatment, and patient and caregiver response to education.

PRESSURE ULCERS

Remember: deep tissue necrosis and loss of tissue volume in the pressure ulcer is disproportionately greater than what appears as the overlying skin defect. This often results in:

- Underestimation of the total problem
- Underestimation of the total length of healing time and the appropriate treatment

Muscle and subcutaneous tissues are highly susceptible to pressure injury from either direct or shearing forces on segmental and perforator arteries while cutaneous vessels often benefit from nearby anastomozing vessels.

Individuals with neurologic, vascular abnormalities as in diabetes mellitus and spinal cord injury have increased susceptibility to pressure injury.

Definition: generally pressure ulcers are local areas of tissue trauma over soft tissue that has been compressed between a bony prominence and any external surface for a prolonged time period. These ulcers are the result of mechanical injury to the skin and underlying tissues.

The National Pressure Ulcer Advisory Panel (NPUAP) has developed the following staging system for determining amount and type of tissue involved in the ulcer:

- Stage I: an observable pressure related alteration in intact skin whose indicators as compared to the adjacent or opposite area on the body may include changes in one or more of the following: skin temperature (warmth or coolness), tissue consistency (firm or boggy feel), and/or sensation (pain, itching). The ulcer appears as a defined area of persistent redness in lightly pigmented skin, whereas in darker skin tones, the ulcer may appear with persistent red, blue, or purple hues (see Figure 3–2.).
- Stage II: partial-thickness skin loss involving epidermis or dermis, or both. The ulcer is superficial and presents clinically as an abrasion, blister, or shallow crater (see Figure 3-3).
- Stage III: full-thickness skin loss involving damage or necrosis of subcutaneous tissue, which may extend down to but not through underlying fascia. The ulcer presents clinically as a deep crater with or without undermining of adjacent tissue (see Figure 3–4).

- Stage IV: full-thickness skin loss with extensive destruction, tissue necrosis, or damage to muscle, bone, or supporting structures (e.g. tendon, joint capsule) (see Figure 3–5).
- Pressure ulcer characteristics
  — Location: most often over bony prominences
  — Size: any
  — Edema: often present in early stages
  — Pain: stage I and II most common
  — Stage I, II, III, or IV
    ▪ With or without necrotic, devitalized tissue
    ▪ With or without exudate
    ▪ Periwound skin often involved
    ▪ Wound edges: vary; may have undermining, tunneling, or hypergranulation
- Patient risk factors for pressure ulcer development:
- Red rest required, especially if chronically ill or obese
- Dehydration
- Diabetes mellitus
- Diminished awareness of pain
- Fractures
- Corticosteroid therapy
- Inadequate nutritional status (especially malnutrition)
- Immunosuppression
- Incontinence (urinary, fecal, or both)
- Mental impairments:
  — Altered consciousness levels
  — Coma
  — Sedation
  — Confusion
  — Alzheimer disease
  — Depression
- Multiple trauma sites or systems

- Paralysis
- Inadequate circulation (venous, arterial, or both)
- Significant obesity or thinness
- History of previous pressure ulcers
- The following risk factors may also be responsible for non-healing or slow healing in any wound type:
- Pressure: immobility, inactivity, and loss of sensory perception affect the duration and intensity of pressure. Individuals who have greater than 50 spontaneous movements a night (in one study) did not develop pressure ulcers while those with 20 or fewer movements developed pressure ulcers.[7]
  - 12–32 mm Hg capillary closing pressure
  - Low intensity over a long time
  - High intensity over a short time
- Common locations
  - Scapula
  - Iliac crest
  - Trochanter
  - Sacrum/coccyx
  - Ischial tuberosities
  - Lateral malleolus
  - Lateral edge of foot
  - Heel (dorsal or lateral aspect, then plantar)
- Protocols for pressure prevention and treatment
  - Pressure reduction
  - Pressure relief
- Turning schedules by patient need, not protocol (only full body change of position completely relieves pressure) (Figures 9–2 and 9–3).
  - 30-degree lateral, not side lying
- Pillow bridging (Figure 9–4)
  - Under legs to elevate heels

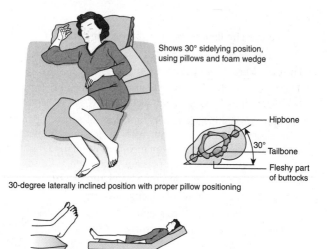

Shows 30° sidelying position, using pillows and foam wedge

Hipbone

30°

Tailbone

Fleshy part of buttocks

30-degree laterally inclined position with proper pillow positioning

Proper heel placement   Head of bed elevation limited to 30° or less

Figure 9–2 Positioning. (From Maklebust JA, Sieggreen M. *Pressure Ulcers Guidelines for Prevention and Nursing Management.* 2nd ed. Springhouse Corp; 1996.)

— Between the ankles
— Between the knees
— Behind the back (some controversy)
— Under the head with neck supported
• Exercise and mobility (active and passive range of motion)
• Do not use donuts or rings or massage to the area
• Restorative nursing program
• Friction: a contributing factor to the development of pressure ulcers and will also prolong healing of any wound. It reduces the tissue tolerance to pressure by abrading and damaging the epidermal and upper dermal skin layers. When friction exists with pressure, ulcers are produced at lower pressure levels.

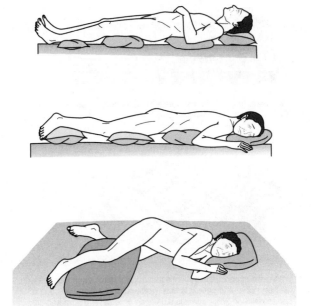

Figure 9–3 Appropriate Positioning. (From Maklebust JA, Sieggreen M. 1996. *Pressure Ulcers Guidelines for Prevention and Nursing Management*. 2nd ed. Springhouse Corp; 1996.)

Friction in conjunction with shear contributes to the development of sacral and/or coccygeal pressure ulcers with patients in a semi-Fowler position.

- Protocols for friction prevention and treatment
  — Skin sealants (skin barrier wipes; alcohol and non-alcohol based)
  — Moisturizers and skin lubricants (high water content)
  — Elbow and heel protectors
  — Corn starch on bed linens; never talcum powder

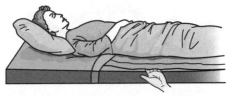

Slide hand (palm up and fingers flat) under support surface, just under
pressure point. Do not flex fingers.

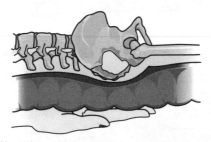

With good support, the patient's bony prominence cannot be felt with
flat hand when the patient is in a "worst-case" position (i.e. head of
bed is elevated 30°, patient is side-lying on greater trochanter, etc.).
Copyright, 1989. Used with permission of Gaymar Industries, Inc.

Figure 9–4 Positioning with Pillow Bridging.

— Appropriate re-positioning techniques
— Restorative nursing program

- Shear: shear acts with a parallel force that causes tissue
  ischemia through lateral blood vessel displacement which
  results in blood flow impediment. It twists and stretches tissue and blood vessels at bony tissue interfaces and therefore
  affects deeper tissue structures and deep blood vessels. Semi-
  Fowler bed position is the most common cause of shear. This
  effect is also the reason many pressure ulcers over a bony
  prominence are substantially larger than the bony prominence over which they occur.

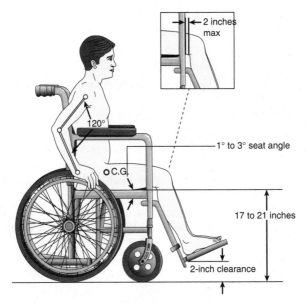

Figure 9–5 Seated Positioning (From Maklebust JA, Sieggreen M. *Pressure Ulcers Guidelines for Prevention and Nursing Management.* 2nd ed. Springhouse Corp; 1996.)

— Gravity plus friction
— Deep fascial level and bony prominences
• Protocols for shear prevention and treatment
    — 30-degree head elevation for short times without allowing the patient to slide down in the bed
    — Foot board
    — Knee gatch
    — Lift sheets
    — Heel protection with dressings, elevated off mattress, and special heel devices; not foam
    — Specialty mattresses and beds; not reimbursable by Medicare unless a wound is present

- — Appropriate re-positioning techniques
- — Restorative nursing program
- Mechanical damage/epidermal stripping
  - — Caregivers (health-care and others)
- Protocols for mechanical damage/epidermal stripping prevention and treatment
  - — Porous tape without tension; apply skin barrier wipe before applying tape if fragile skin is present
  - — Careful adhesive removal using the push-pull technique with all adhesives
  - — Skin sealants: skin barrier wipes; alcohol and non-alcohol based
  - — Other securing methods such as Montgomery straps, non-allergic tape, hydrocolloid under tape, and stretch net dressings
- Moisture: removes protective skin oils from the skin therefore creating more friable skin. It also interacts with friction.
  - — Mild to moderate moisture (diaphoresis, fecal or urinary incontinence, wound exudate); shearing force and friction increase with moisture at these levels.
    - ▪ Incontinence exposes the skin to excess moisture as well as chemical damage.
      - ○ Evaluate cause of urinary incontinence which may be dietary, mechanical, environmental, or physical
      - ○ Bladder training program
    - ▪ Fecal incontinence adds to the risk stated above by adding bacteria and bowel enzymes.
      - ○ Evaluate cause of fecal incontinence which may be dietary, mechanical, environmental or physical
  - — Constant moisture causes maceration—waterlogging of the tissues—which softens connective tissue therefore it becomes more prone to erosion of the epidermis
- Protocols for moisture prevention and treatment

- — Absorbent powders, never talcum powder
- — Skin sealants skin barrier wipes; alcohol and nonalcohol based
- — Dressing changes as necessary
- — Use of cotton materials in skin folds
- — Restorative nursing program
- — CNA/CHHA plan of care
- Mobility
  - — Longer wound healing with less exercise/mobility
- Protocols for immobility prevention and treatment
  - — Encourage independence in all activities
  - — AROM with all dependent activities
  - — Specific exercises
  - — PT/OT referral as indicated
  - — Restorative nursing program
- Blood pressure (B/P)
  - — Systolic below 100
  - — Diastolic below 60
- Protocols for blood pressure treatment
  - — Treat cause and prevention; teach B/P taking
  - — Include B/P on CHHA/CNA plan of care
  - — Diet and fluid log
  - — Medication log
  - — Pre and Post activity B/P
  - — Consider dietitian referral
- Elevated temperature
  - — Especially in the elderly
- Protocols for treatment of elevated temperature
  - — Manage symptoms
  - — Treat cause and prevention (evaluate hydration status)
  - — Include temperature on CHHA/CNA plan of care

— Diet and fluid log
— Dietitian referral
— Medication log
• Medications

These medications prolong or stop wound healing

— Evaluate all medications (efficacy)
— Corticosteroids (withhold for 4 to 5 days after ulcer appearance if possible)
— Antibacterials
— Antihypertensives
— Analgesics
— Antidepressants
— Antihistamines
• Tobacco smoking/use
— Higher incidence and increased time for healing with per numbers of packs per day (pressure and other wound incidence as well as slow/non healing)
• Protocols for tobacco cessation
— Educate and support efforts at reduction and quitting
— Provide literature
• Psychological status
— Motivation
— Emotional energy
• Emotional stress
• Protocols for improving psychological status in pressure ulcers and other chronic wounds
— Encouragement and support
— Relaxation techniques
— Activity
— MSW and chaplain referral
— Psychiatric referral
— Restorative nursing program for exercises

Body Malfunctions: Plan of Care Development

- Evaluate every wounded client for these and focus on treatment, stabilization, and prevention:
- Respiratory system: oxygen deficits; carbon dioxide excesses
  - OT referral for energy conservation
  - Restorative nursing program
  - Pulse oximetry (part of POC)
  - Medication management systems
  - MSW referral for psychosocial interventions, long term planning
- Cardiovascular system: circulation and perfusion to and from wounded area; impaired waste removal; bleeding deficiencies
  - Restorative nursing program
  - OT referral for ADLs and energy conservation
  - Home rehabilitation program (CHHAs)
  - Medication management systems
  - Compression therapy at wound sites (vascular)
  - MSW referral for psychosocial interventions, long term planning
- Gastrointestinal system: malabsorption; acidity and alkalinity of secretions, excretions
  - CHHA/CNA POC includes nutrition and meal preparation
  - Restorative nursing program (bowel retraining)
  - Dietitian referral
  - SLP/OT referral for swallowing evaluation
  - MSW referral for reduced costs of food, psychosocial interventions (especially with incontinence)
- Musculoskeletal system: immobility; position awareness
  - PT/OT referral
  - CNA POC

— Home rehabilitation program (CHHAs)
— Restorative nursing program
— MSW referral for DME costs, psychosocial interventions, long term planning

• Genitourinary system: moisture and chemical irritation; faulty collagen deposition; impaired waste removal
  — Correct barrier product use
    ▪ Petrolatum based moisture barriers
    ▪ Zinc oxide based barriers
    ▪ Skin barrier wipes; alcohol and non-alcohol based
    ▪ Hydrocolloid on wounds as appropriate
  — Avoid adult plastic diapers whenever possible
  — Avoid continuous Foley catheterization of bladder except in cases of retention. Foley catheter may be necessary for short term (2 to 4 weeks) if the wounded skin cannot be kept free of urinary incontinence in any other manner
  — CHHA/CNA referral
  — Restorative nursing program for bladder retraining
  — OT referral for ADLs, devices
  — ET referral for containment devices, skin treatment
  — MSW referral for costs of products, psychosocial interventions especially with incontinence

• Neurological system: impaired awareness and sensation
  — PT/OT referral
  — Home rehabilitation program
  — Restorative nursing program
  — MSW referral for costs of products and durable medical equipment (DME), psychosocial interventions, long term planning
  — Speech language pathologist (SLP) referral for communication and or swallowing

— Evaluate all skin folds especially on affected limbs for rashes and tears

  ▪ Use anti-fungal topically such as Lotrimin 1% with physician order
  ▪ Acetic acid 0.25% on fungal rash; cools the itching and burning
  ▪ Do not cover rashes with dressings. If clothing is necessary in the rash area advised to wear 100% cotton. The clothing and bedding must be washed in hot water and white household vinegar added to the rinse cycle (1 to 2 cups for large loads). If using antifungals for foot rashes, the shoes must be cleansed with acetic acid solution, allowed to dry in direct sunlight and re-cleansed after every use. Use of an over the counter antifungal foot powder in the shoes is also advisable.

• Endocrine system: infection; retarded healing; basement membrane thickening

  — Evaluate blood sugars
  — MSW referral for costs of products and DME, psychosocial interventions, long term planning
  — Diabetes nurse specialist referral
  — Dietitian referral

Additional Risk Factors that Delay Wound Healing

• Heredity
• Malignancies
• Substance abuse
• Radiation
• Chemotherapy
• Foreign bodies
• Inability to control, reduce, and eliminate other risk factors
• Iatrogenic factors

Pressure Ulcer Treatment

- AHCPR (now AHRQ) guidelines (becoming dated)
- Prevention
- Timely reassessments and evaluations of treatments
- Skin cleansing
- Minimize skin drying
- Eliminate and minimize massage of affected areas
- Eliminate and minimize pressure; evaluate all support surfaces for 'bottoming out' at each visit and correct when present
- Eliminate and minimize friction and shear
- Eliminate and minimize exposure to incontinence, exudate, and perspiration
- Assess and treat: all risk factors, pain, and psychological states
- Educate caregivers and patient on prevention, signs and symptoms to report, and treatment
- Healthpoint product information obtained from www.health-point.com.
- Accuzyme Papain-Urea Debriding Ointment
- Panafil Debriding, deoderizing and healing ointment"

Clinical Alert
Remember that pressure ulcers may occur in many areas of the body although generally they are local areas of tissue trauma over soft tissue where pressure has compressed one area of tissue between a bony prominence and any external surface for a prolonged time period.

KEY CONCEPTS

Whenever evaluating or treating a suspected or previously diagnosed pressure ulcer:

Remember:

1. Loss of tissue volume and deep tissue necrosis in the pressure ulcer is disproportionately greater than what appears as overlying skin damage. This may result in:
   — Underestimation of the total length of healing time and the appropriate treatment
   — Underestimation of the total problem

2. Muscle and subcutaneous tissues are highly susceptible to pressure injury from either direct or shearing forces on segmental and perforator arteries while cutaneous vessels often benefit from nearby anastomizing vessels.

3. Individuals with neurological, vascular abnormalities such as diabetes mellitus and spinal cord injury have increased susceptibility to pressure injury.

4. The health-care provider should assess clients for the risk of developing pressure ulcers using a validated tool such as the Braden Risk Assessment Scale for the development of Pressure Ulcers or the Norton Pressure Ulcer Risk Assessment Scale. And plan individualized treatment based on the particular client's needs and risk factors.

- Evaluate every wounded client for risk factors that delay wound healing and focus on treatment, stabilization, and prevention
- Respiratory system: oxygen deficits; carbon dioxide excesses
- OT referral for energy conservation
- Restorative nursing program including CNA
- Pulse oximetry (part of POC)
- Medication management systems
- MSW referral for psychosocial interventions, long term planning
- Cardiovascular system: circulation and perfusion to and from wounded area; impaired waste removal; bleeding deficiencies
- Restorative nursing program including CNA
- OT referral for ADLs and energy conservation

- Home rehabilitation program (CHHAs)
- Medication management systems
- Compression therapy at wound sites (vascular)
- MSW referral for psychosocial interventions, long term planning
- Gastrointestinal system: malabsorption; acidity and alkalinity of secretions, excretions
- CHHA/CNA POC may include nutrition and meal preparation
- Restorative nursing program for bowel retraining including CNA
- Dietitian referral
- SLP/OT referral for swallowing evaluation
- MSW referral for reduced costs of food and psychosocial interventions, especially with incontinence
- Musculoskeletal system: immobility; position awareness
- PT/OT referral
- CNA POC
- Home rehabilitation program (CHHAs)
- Restorative nursing program including CNA
- MSW referral for DME costs, psychosocial interventions, long term planning
- Genitourinary system: moisture and chemical irritation; faulty collagen deposition; impaired waste removal
- Correct barrier product use
- Petrolatum based moisture barriers
- Zinc Oxide based barriers
- Skin barrier wipes; alcohol and non-alcohol based
- Hydrocolloid on wounds as appropriate
- Avoid adult plastic diapers whenever possible
- Avoid continuous Foley catheterization of bladder except in cases of retention. Foley catheter may be necessary for short term (2 to 4 weeks) if the wounded skin cannot be kept free of urinary incontinence in any other manner

- CHHA/CNA referral
- Restorative nursing program of bladder retraining including CNA
- OT referral for ADLs, devices
- WOC nurse referral for containment devices, skin treatment
- MSW referral for costs of products, psychosocial interventions especially with incontinence
- Neurological system: impaired awareness and sensation
- PT/OT referral
- Home rehabilitation program
- Restorative nursing program including CNA
- MSW referral for costs of products and DME, psychosocial interventions, long term planning
- SLP referral for communication and or swallowing.
- Evaluates all skin folds especially on affected limbs for rashes and tears
- Use anti-fungal topically such as Lotrimin® 1% with physician order
- Acetic acid 0.25% on fungal rash; cools the itching and burning
- Do not cover rashes with dressings. If clothing is necessary in the rash area, advise to wear 100% breathable cotton. The clothing and bedding must be washed in hot water and white household vinegar added to the rinse cycle (1 to 2 cups for large loads).

If using antifungals for foot rashes, the shoes must be cleansed with acetic acid solution and allowed to dry in direct sunlight and re-cleansed after every use. Use of an over the counter antifungal foot powder in the shoes is also advisable.

- Endocrine system: infection; retarded healing, basement membrane thickening
- Evaluate blood sugars
- MSW referral for costs of products and DME, psychosocial interventions, long term planning

- Diabetes nurse specialist referral
- Dietitian referral
- Additional risk factors that increase risk for non or prolonged healing
- Heredity
- Malignancies
- Substance abuse
- Radiation
- Chemotherapy
- Foreign bodies
- Inability to control, reduce, eliminate other risk factors
- Iatrogenic factors
- Pressure ulcer treatment
- Prevention
- Timely reassessments and evaluations of treatments
- Skin cleansing
- Minimize skin drying
- Eliminate and minimize massage of affected areas
- Eliminate and minimize pressure; evaluate all support surfaces for 'bottoming out' at each encounter and correct when present
- Eliminate and minimize friction and shear
- Eliminate and minimize exposure to incontinence, exudate, and perspiration
- Assess and treat: all risk factors, pain, psychological states
- Educate caregivers and client on prevention, signs and symptoms to report, and treatment

SUPPORT SURFACES

These surfaces are a major component of treatment and prevention of pressure ulcers and are used to control pressure. Some surfaces reduce friction, shear, control moisture, and inhibit bacterial proliferation. These devices are available in a multitude of shapes and sizes for use on beds, in chairs, and on limbs.

- Pressure reduction or pressure relief?
  - The ideal would be visualization of soft tissue on the device with results indicating no deforming of the soft tissue while on the device. This is not practical in most clinical settings and therefore it is the responsibility of the health-care provider to be aware of the type of available devices, the appropriate selection for each client, and client and caregiver education regarding use and management of the device.
    - Reduction devices lower the pressure on a specific surface below the pressure that would be experienced without the device.
    - Relief devices (very few are available and all statements about this should be carefully evaluated) relieve pressure on a specific surface by reducing the level of pressure to below capillary closing pressures.
  - Dynamic or static?

Dynamic surfaces alternate inflation and deflation, some accomplish this with only the force of the individual's breathing others may require stronger patient movements, and some are programmed to change with the passage of time.

Static surfaces maintain a constant inflation (by gel, foam, water) that molds to the body surface spreading the pressure load over a large (rather than small as in pressure ulcer development) area.

Types of Devices

- Foam overlays: commonly used for pressure reduction. Important characteristics of the device:
  - Base height and thickness (height from base to top). This varies with various products even from the same manufacturer.

— Two (2) inches of medical grade foam are for comfort only and do not reduce or relieve pressure.

— Three to four inches may reduce pressure if the patient is not overweight and surface is medical grade.

— Important to validate what loads (weight amount) the manufacturer is allowed to state the device is capable of holding for either reduction or relief.

— Density of the foam material (ability to support patient's weight).

— Indentation load deflection (ILD) (compressibility, conformability of foam and foam's ability to distribute the mechanical load).

— Some foam devices are medical grade foam while others are not and therefore each device should be carefully evaluated to meet the individual client's needs and use.

— Contours (the surface description i.e. convoluted, slashed, flat, or textured).

— Health-care provider responsible for evaluation of client's overall body weight, distribution on the support surface, and for ordering a surface that provides either prevention or appropriate treatment of wounds.

• Static air-filled overlays: interconnected cells in the device are interconnected when inflated usually with an air blower.

— Some devices are medical grade foam while others are not and therefore each device should be carefully evaluated to meet the individual client's needs and use.

— Available for chair or bed use, for short or long term use.

— Vast majority reduce pressure, a few market pressure relief.

— Proper inflation is an absolute necessity.

• Alternating air-filled mattress overlays: inflation and deflation occurs on an alternating basis with the intent of preventing constant pressure against the skin.

— Some devices are medical grade foam while others are not and therefore each device should be carefully evaluated to meet the individual client's needs and use.

— May enhance blood flow

— Proper inflation is an absolute necessity

- Gel or water-filled mattress overlays:

  — Some gel devices are medical grade foam while others are not and therefore each device should be carefully evaluated to meet the individual client's needs and use.

  — These overlays offer pressure reduction and are easy to clean while requiring little maintenance.

  — Gel is also used as a mattress replacement in some settings.

  — Gel-filled cushions are also available for chairs.

  — Most gel devices cause temperature to increase over time with skin/client contact and therefore may increase the surface temperature during unrelieved periods of unrelieved sitting. Client's must be taught to reposition frequently (usually every 15 minutes) to reduce the negative effects of this temperature increase.

  — Most gel devices are nonporous and this increases the relative humidity of the skin. Clients must be taught to reposition frequently (usually every 15 minutes) to reduce the negative effects of this moisture increase.

  — Mattress replacements are also available. These may include foam, gel, combination fillings, and air.

  — Most are covered with bacteriostatic material but few studies exist that attest to the long term efficacy and ability of these coverings to control infection.

- Low air-loss mattress replacements: many of these are supported directly on the bed frame, replacing the existing mattress.

  — Consist of connected, air-filled compartments or cushions throughout the device. Each of these areas is inflated to a specific pressure based on the client's height, weight, and weight distribution. An air pump circulates a continuous air flow through the device.

— Some products individualize each of the compartments within the device to adjust for head, trunk, and foot areas.

— Some products are alternating while others have pulsating pressure features.

— Most are easy to set up and take down and are therefore used in a variety of health-care settings.

— Most come with waterproof coverings designed to allow air to pass through; these do not usually create wound dehydration but the wound/s must be consistently evaluated for this potential.

• Low air-loss specialty beds: these beds provide a more even distribution of the patient's weight over a sequence of air filled pillows. The source of the air is a pumping motor that allows dry air to flow between the patient and the surface. This dry air controls moisture and heat buildup. It is important to know the patient's height, weight, and (often) the body-fat distribution to obtain the appropriate bed.

• Air-fluidized specialty beds: a pump distributes air through silicone-coated microspheres that are separated from the patient by a monofilament sheet. The general feeling is one of floating.

— These beds are often very heavy and may cause the wound/s to dry out.

— For some clients this type of device makes repositioning difficult and/or impossible without the assistance of at least one other ably bodied person.

— These devices create the greatest immersion for the client; however it must be remembered that repositioning is still required when using one of these devices.

Goal of appropriate bed surface and device:

• Prevention or treatment of Stage I or II with one sleep surface impaired

— May use alternating pressure pad, 6 inches or greater medical grade foam

— NO donuts or rings

- Treatment of stage III or IV with one sleep surface impaired:

— May use static mattress or overlay or dynamic mattress or overlay; limit sitting time if wound on ischial tuberosity

— NO donuts or rings

- Treatment of flap or graft, burn or stage II with two or three sleep surfaces impaired:

— May use dynamic, low air loss, or air fluidized mattress on bed, reduce amount of sitting time if wounds are on ischial tuberosities

— NO donuts or rings

- Treatment of stage III or IV with two or three sleep surfaces impaired:

— May use low air loss or air fluidized bed; limit amount of sitting time

— NO donuts or rings

- Any patient who will be sitting for periods of time and has a wound on a sitting surface or is at risk of developing one requires an appropriate pressure reduction device on all sitting surfaces.

- ALL support surfaces should be evaluated for 'bottoming out' at each visit and every day or shift and the caregiver and patient educated in how to check this.

- Reimbursement for support surfaces in home health:

- Covered under Medicare Part B (DME)

- Must be multiple stage IIs, Stage III or IV pressure ulcer

- Must be located on trunk of body

- Patient must be living in his or her permanent residence

- Positioning and Seating (Figures 9–2 through 9–5)

- Greater risk with sitting than lying down

— Gravitational force creates greater body weight over smaller surface with seated activities than when flat in bed because more surface to disperse pressures when flat in bed.

- Emphasis:
  — Posture
  — Alignment
  — Avoidance of sitting on pressure ulcers or reddened areas
  — Anterior thighs
    ▪ Horizontal
      ○ Distributes weight evenly along posterior surfaces
      ○ If knees are higher than hips; body weight is shifted to ischial tuberosities that increases pressure risk
  — Reduce risk of pressure on ischial tuberosities by keeping neutral position of:
    ▪ Ankles
    ▪ Elbows
    ▪ Forearms
    ▪ Wrists
  — Knees should not rub together; keep them separated
    ▪ Keep seat angle with knees no higher than buttocks to keep ischial and sacral pressure at a minimum to reduce incidence of pressure ulcers

- Repositioning
  — Every 15 minutes
  — If patient has the upper body strength, educate to do push-ups to re-establish buttocks and sacral blood flow every 15 minutes.
  — If patient does not have upper body strength, educate
    ▪ To lean forward toward the thighs to reduce pressure over the ischial tuberosities (from 189 mm Hg to 34 mm Hg and on the ischium from 114 mm Hg to 33 mm HG in one study.[8]

- Chair sitting for those unable to reposition themselves should be limited to 1 hour at a time, then the patient placed back in bed.[9]

— All patients in chairs who are at risk should have pressure reduction devices in the chairs in which they are sitting at all times.

— All pressure reduction devices for sitting surfaces should be evaluated for 'bottoming out' minimally at least each shift or twice daily.

— Patients and caregivers require education in how to perform this and return demonstrations should be documented in every level of care before discharge to the next level of care.

— Additionally, for all support devices the patient and a caregiver must minimally be knowledgeable concerning:

- How a device functions, or is intended to function
- What is the cost or share of cost for the device
- Where the device is coming from
- Who is responsible for maintaining the device
- Who and how to contact if there are any problems with the function of the device
- Who is responsible for maintenance of any accoutrements of pads, covers, buzzers, and whistles
- Where the booklet is kept explaining how the device works
- When and how long the warranty lasts
- How, who, and when a device is to be cleaned

— Some companies that provide some or all of these product types:

- Chestnut Ridge
- Gaymar
- DeRoyal
- EHOB, Inc
- Gaymar

- Hill-Rom
- Huntleigh
- KCI
- Keen Mobility
- Mason Medical Products
- Medline
- Span-America
- Tempur-Pedic

— Medicare coverage for these products changes overtime and can be accessed at

http://www.medicare.gov

PRESSURE ULCER TREATMENT RELATIVE TO STAGE

Remember to educate all CNAs and CHHAs on the following aspects:

Stage I

- Inspection of all bony prominences during waking hours every shift, twice daily, or more often
- Pressure reduction with turning schedule every 2 hours
- Heels off of mattress while in bed
- NO massaging of the ulcer or periwound skin
- Requires dressing only if in an area of moisture or friction i.e. incontinence or heels
- Apply either a non-adherent, protective dressing such as Kendall Preppies®, 3M No-Sting Barrier Wipe®, Non-woven gauze, Adaptic® (use with caution)
- Use extreme care with any cleansing of ulcer
- Instruct patient and family in basic skin care and repositioning while in bed and while seated (Figures 9–4 and 9–5)
- Avoid use of diapers if ulcer is in area of incontinence whenever possible

— Appropriate lifting and positioning techniques
— Avoid use of soap to all dry skin areas. Lotion may be used in bath water.
— Apply moisturizers BID to entire body
— Inspect and evaluate shoe gear for evidence of improper fit

Stage II:

- Inspection of all bony prominences during waking hours every shift, twice daily, or more often
- Pressure reduction with turning schedule every 2 hours
- Heels off of mattress while in bed
- Foot cradle if ulcer is on foot/toe/heel
- NO massaging of the ulcer or periwound skin
- Instruct patient and family in basic skin care and repositioning while in bed and while seated
- Appropriate lifting and positioning techniques
- Avoid use of soap to all dry skin areas. Lotion may be used in bath water.
- Apply moisturizers BID to entire body
- Inspect/evaluate shoe gear for evidence of improper fit
- Evaluate nutritional and hydration status, change plan of care as appropriate
- Ulcer treatment (NOT heel blisters):
- Cleanse gently with Normal Saline (NS)
- Cover with hydrocolloid, 3M Tegasorb®
- Appropriate application of any hydrocolloid requires that a minimum of 1.0 cm of intact skin is at the wound edge is under the dressing.
  — Change every 3 to 5 days and prn leaking, peeling, or contamination with incontinence.
- Heel blister treatment:
- If skin on heel is intact no dressing is necessary if heel is elevated off mattress and leg is elevated when up in chair.
- If skin is open:

- Cleanse gently with NS
- Cover with non-stick, non-woven gauze, or Telfa® and dry dressing every day or Adaptic® (use with caution) and dry gauze every day.
- Instruct client/family (when discharge to home is planned) in:
- Proper handwashing
- Signs/symptoms of infection to report
- Wound care
- Nutrition and hydration principles
- Prevention of additional pressure ulcers
- Proper transfer techniques

Stage III:

- Inspection of all bony prominences during waking hours (every shift/BID or more often)
- Pressure reduction with turning schedule every 2 hours
- Heels off of mattress while in bed
- Foot cradle if ulcer is on foot/toe/heel
- **NO** massaging of the ulcer or periwound skin
- Instruct client/family in basic skin care and repositioning while in bed and while seated
  — Appropriate lifting and positioning techniques
  — Avoid use of soap to all dry skin areas. Lotion may be used in bath water.
  — Apply moisturizers BID to entire body
  — Inspect/evaluate shoe gear for evidence of improper fit
  — Evaluate nutritional and hydration status, change plan of care as appropriate
  — Limit time up in chair if ulcer is on sitting surface (usually 1 hour; 1–3 times per day)
  — Ulcer treatment:
  — Clean gently with NS (wound cleanser with surfactant Kendall CuraClenz® if exudate is tenacious)

— Apply hydrogel (for example: Smith&Nephew Solosite® product with preservative or Intrasite® gel product without preservative) directly to wound or to primary dressing and avoid product contact with intact periwound skin

— Cover with dry dressing

— Change every day or twice daily depending on amount of exudate

— If large amounts of exudate (more than 50% of secondary dressing is saturated in less than 24 hours) do not use hydrogel but apply calcium alginate (for example: Hollister Restore Calcicare®).

— Keep alginate in contact with wounded skin only to prevent desiccation.

— Cover with dry dressing

— Change daily or every other day or less often dependent on amount of exudate.

* Instruct client and family when discharge to home is planned in:

* Proper handwashing

* Signs and symptoms of infection to report

* Wound care

* Nutrition and hydration principles

* Prevention of additional pressure ulcers

* Proper transfer techniques

Stage IV:

* Inspection of all bony prominences during waking hours (every shift or more often)

* Pressure reduction with turning schedule every 2 hours

* Heels off mattress while in bed

* Foot cradle if ulcer is on foot/toe/heel

* NO massaging of the ulcer or periwound skin

* Instruct patient and family in basic skin care and repositioning while in bed and while seated

— Appropriate lifting and positioning techniques

- Avoid use of soap to all dry skin areas. Lotion may be used in bath water.
- Apply moisturizers BID to entire body
- Inspect/evaluate shoe gear for evidence of improper fit
- Evaluate nutritional and hydration status, change plan of care as appropriate
- Limit time up in chair if ulcer is on sitting surface (usually 1 hour; 1–3 times per day)

• Ulcer treatment:

- Clean gently with NS (wound cleanser with surfactant, (for example: Kendall CuraClenz if exudate is tenacious)
- Apply hydrogel (for example Smith&Nephew Solosite® product with preservative or Intrasite gel (product without preservative) directly to wound or to primary dressing and avoid product contact with intact periwound skin
- Cover with dry dressing
- Change every day or twice daily dependent on amount of exudate
- If large amounts of exudate (more than 50% of secondary dressing is saturated in less than 24 hours) do not use hydrogel but apply calcium alginate (for example Hollister Restore Calcicare).
- Keep alginate in contact with wounded skin only to prevent desiccation.
- Cover with dry dressing
- Change daily or every other day.

• Instruct client and family when discharge to home or transfer to lower level of care is planned in:

• Proper handwashing

• Signs and symptoms of infection to report

• Wound care

• Nutrition and hydration principles

• Prevention of additional pressure ulcers

• Proper transfer techniques

REFERENCES

1. Baranoski S, Ayello E *Wound Care Essentials Practice Principles*. Philadelphia, PA: Lippincott Williams & Wilkins; 2004.
2. Committee on the Control of Surgical Infections of the Committee on Pre- and Postoperative Care of the American College of Surgeons. *Manual on Control of Infection in Surgical Patients*. Philadelphia, PA: Lippincott Williams & Wilkens; 1976.
3. Mertz PM, Ovington LG. Wound Healing Microbiology. *Dermatology Clinics*. Oct 1993;11(4):739–47.
4. Winter GD. Formation of the scab and the rate of epithelialization of superficial wounds in the skin of young domestic pigs. *Nature*. 1962;193:293–94.
5. Kim YC, et al. Efficacy of hydrocolloid occlusive dressing technique in decubitus ulcer treatment: A comparative study. *Yonsei Med J*. 1996;37:181–185.
6. Ovington L. Hanging wet to dry dressings out to dry. *Advances in Skin & Wound Care*. Mar-Apr 2002;15(2):79–86.
7. Exton-Smith & Sherwin. Monitoring the mobility of patients in bed. *Medical and Biological Engineering and Computing*. 1985;23(5):466–468.
8. Maklebust JA, Sieggreen M. *Pressure Ulcers Guidelines for Prevention and Nursing Managemen.t* 2nd ed. Springhouse, PA: Springhouse Corp; 1996.
9. AHCPR 1992 Prevention and treatment of pressure ulcers. Pressure Ulcers in Adults: Prediction and Prevention Clinical Practice Guideline Number 3. Available online at: http://www.ncbi.nlm.nih.gov/books/bv.fcgi?rid=hstat2.chapter.4409. Accessed July 20,2008.

SUGGESTED READING

Bryant, Ruth A. 2000. *Acute and Chronic Wounds 2ⁿᵈ ed*. Mosby , St. Louis, MO.

Cullum N, McInnes E, Bell-Syer SEM, Legood R. Support surfaces for pressure ulcer prevention. *Cochrane Database of Systematic Reviews* 1998, Issue 1. Art. No: CD001735. DOI: 10.1002/14651858.CD001735.pub2. This version first published online: January 26. 1998 Date of last subtantive update: May 20. 2004.

Cunningham D. Treating venous insufficiency ulcers with soft silicone dressings. *Ostomy Wound Manage.* 2005;51(11A suppl):21–22.

Cuzzell, Janice. 1990 Clues: Bruised, Torn Skin. *AJN March 1990* pp. 16–17.

Ennis, William J & Meneses, Patricio. 2000 Wound Healing at the Local Level: The Stunned Wound. *Ostomy/Wound Management January 2000 Supplement V 46 Issue 1A pp. 39S–48S*

Falanga, Vincent. 2002. Wound Bed Preparation and the Role of Enzymes: A Case for Multiple Actions of Therapeutic Agents. *Wounds 14(2): 47–57.*

Hall, John C. 2000. *Sauer's Manual of Skin Diseases* 8th ed. Lippincott Williams & Wilkins Philadelphia, PA.

Harker J. Influences on patient adherence with compression hosiery. *J Wound Care.* 2000;9(8):379–382.

Hess, Cathy T. 1998 *Wound Care* 2nd ed. Springhouse Corp. Springhouse, PA.

Hess, Cathy T. 2000 *Wound Care* 3rd ed. Springhouse Corp. Springhouse, PA.

Kim JS, et al. Antimicrobial effects of silver nanoparticles. *Nanomedicine.* 2007;3(1):95–101.

Krasner D. Caring for a person experiencing chronic wound pain. In: Krasner DL, Rodeheaver GT, Sibbald RG (eds). *Chronic Wound Care: A Clinical Source Book for Healthcare Professionals (3rd ed).* Wayne, Pa: HMP Communications;2001;79–89.

Neil JA, Munjas BA. Living with a chronic wound: The voices of sufferers. *Ostomy Wound Manage.* 2000;46(5):28–38.

Papadopopoulos, A. et al. 1999. Motivation and compliance in wound management. *Journal of Wound Care October. Vol. .8. No. 9. Pp. 467–69.*

Payne, Regina L. et al 1993 Defining and classifying skin tears: Need for a common language. *Ostomy/Wound Management V39 (5)*

Petro, J. 1992 Ethical and Psychosocial Considerations of Wound Management. *Decubitus pp. 22–25 January 1992.*

Rhinehart, Emily. 2001. Infection Control in Home Care. *Emerg. Infect. Dis. 7(2): 2001.* www.medscape.com

Seidel, Henry, Ball, Jane, Dains, Joyce, and Benedict G.William. 1999 *Mosby's Guide to Physical Examination* 4th Edition. Mosby Inc. St Louis, MO.

Stalano-Coico et al 2000. Wound Fluids: A Reflection of the State of Healing. *Ostomy/Wound Management January 2000 Supplement V 46 Issue 1A pp. 85S–93S.*

Sussman, C & Bates-Jensen, B 1998 *Wound Care A Collaborative Practice Manual for Physical Therapists and Nurses.* Aspen Publications, Gaithersburg, MD.

Support Systems International, Inc. 1993 *The Skin, Module 1.* Hillenbrand, Charleston, SC.

Swartz, Mark. 1998 *Textbook of Physical Diagnosis History and Examination 3rd edition.* W.B. Saunders Co Philadelphia, PA.

Tierney, L, McPhee, S, and Papadakis, M. 1998 *Current Medical Diagnosis and Treatment 37th edition.* Appleton & Lange, Stamford, CT.

White, Marguerite W. et al 1994 Skin Tears in Frail Elders: A Practical Approach to Prevention. *Geriatric Nursing V 15 #2 pp. 95-99.*

Wientjes KA. Mind-body techniques in wound healing. *Ostomy Wound Manage.* 2002;48(11):62–67.

WOCN Guidance on OASIS Skin and Wound Status MO Items – Spring 2001. http://www. deroyal.com/Wound_Care

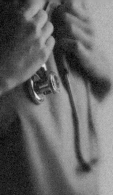

Chapter 10

SKIN ASSESSMENT AND DOCUMENTATION

🔑 KEY POINTS

- Skin anatomy and physiology.
- Ethical concepts to be considered in providing wound management to clients/patients.
- Components of patient privacy when receiving wound care.
- Functions of the skin including the layer and cells that perform each function.
- Functions of fibroblasts, macrophages, and mast cells during homeostasis.
- Effects of aging on the skin and relevance when providing wound care.
- Components of the integumentary history and physical for clients/patients with wounds.
- Expected skin findings in older adults.
- Types and application of tape and/or adhesive used in general and in specific instances of wound care.

SKIN ANATOMY AND PHYSIOLOGY

The skin is the largest body organ; it represents approximately 15% of total body weight and utilizes 20% of body's protein. The two layers of the skin are the epidermis and dermis (subcutaneous layer is not actually a skin layer but is usually presented in discussions on the skin). Accessories to the skin are the hair, sweat glands, and nails.

Thickness of the skin varies from one-fiftieth of an inch in the eyelids to one-third inch on the palms and soles. Texture, color, amount of hair, and appearance differ among races, individuals, between males and females, and at different ages.

Functions of skin

- Protection
- Environmental sensing organ
- Water retention
- Thermoregulation
- Immune response

- Production of vitamin D
- Emotional response

Layers of skin

- Epidermis
  — Stratified epithelial tissue
  — No blood vessels
  — Receives nutrition and oxygen via diffusion for the dermal capillaries
  — Five layers from the inside to the outside are: (1) stratum germinativum (also called "stratum basale"); (2) stratum spinosum; (3) stratum granulosum; (4) stratum lucidum; (5) stratumcorneum
    - Stratum germinativum: basal layer that actively proliferates.
    - One-cell thick generates keratinocytes by constant mitosis.
    - Keratinocytes produce the protein keratin that imparts durability to the epidermis.
    - Keratinocytes progress from the basal layer to the outer layer in 4 to 6 weeks and keratin slowly evolves during this time.
    - Specialized cell wall structures, desmosomes, connect adjacent keratinocytes to provide adhesion at each layer during the progression upward.
    - Stratum spinosum and stratum germinativum create granules:
      ○ Keratinohyalin
      ○ Proteins
      ○ Lipids
    These are released into spaces between cells to form ground substance. The ground substance is responsible for the selective permeability of the epidermis.
    - Cell membrane transformation occurs in these layers. This transformation in the epidermis provides that layer

with the ability to resist degradation from various solvents.

— Stratum corneum:
  - Cornified, dead, flat cells including15 facial regions and more than 100 regions on palms and soles.
  - Prevents entrance of toxic substances and microorganisms.
  - Prevents water loss and is almost impermeable to water.
  - Desquamation: cells break apart due to desmosome destruction causes cell shedding.

— Epidermal cells
  - Langerhans: immune system and the first defense line against environmental antigens.
  - Melanocytes: melanosomes synthesize melanin, which is released into the extracellular space and taken upward by keratinocytes.
    - Absorbs light as a protection against solar radiation and is distributed throughout all layers of the epidermis.

— Dermal-epidermal junction formed by a basement membrane between the epidermis and the dermis.
  - Collagen in a honeycomb type form that provides a framework with tensile strength and elasticity in which epithelial cells of the epidermis become firmly attached.
  - Filters, allowing some substances through and excluding others.
  - Disruption of the basement membrane is associated with the formation of blisters.

- Dermis
  — Connective tissue that forms an interlocking web of fibrous proteins and nonfibrous ground substance.
  — Contains:
  — Cells
  — Skin appendages
  — Nerves
  — Vascular system elements

- Functions:
  - — Epidermal nutrition
  - — Protection from mechanical injury and microorganisms
  - — Environmental sensing organ
  - — Thermoregulation

- Dermal regions: papillary and reticular
  - — Papillary dermis: a narrow area immediately beneath the basement membrane.
    - ▪ Microscopically resembles an egg carton, three-dimensional structure.
    - ▪ Capillary loops from the papillary blood vessel plexis extend up toward the epidermis and are primarily responsible for epidermal nutrition, response to injury, and thermoregulation.
  - — Reticular dermis: larger component forming the majority of the dermal layer.
    - ▪ Cell density is less than in papillary region.
    - ▪ Contains: (deep structures)
      - ○ Hair follicles
      - ○ Sweat glands
      - ○ Collagen, reticulin, and elastin fibers in a framework that resists stretch but not uniformly. Cleavage lines are subtle differences in fiber orientation that surgeons often try to follow when making incisions parallel rather than across them to reduce scar tissue.

- Dermal cells
  - — Fibroblasts: synthesis, breakdown, and remodeling of connective tissue matrix in a process called fibroplasia. Proliferate whenever skin is damaged and represent a major force in healing the skin.
    - ▪ Proteins collagen and elastin provide the bulk, density, tensile strength, elasticity, and compliance of skin. Fibroblasts synthesize these proteins.

- Tensile strength: resistance to stretch.
- Elasticity: ability to return to original state following stretch.
- Compliance: ability to bend.
- All the above enable skin to move and stretch as well as protect skin from shear and friction.

— Macrophages: cells from bone marrow that occur in the blood as monocytes and migrate into tissues.

- Phagocytize bacteria, dead cell fragments, and other debris.
- Control infection through ingestion of bacteria.
- Excrete ascorbic acid, hydrogen peroxide, and lactic acid (body sends more macrophages at this time).
- Secrete angiogenesis growth factor that stimulates budding of endothelial cells from damaged blood vessels.
- Occur in all phases of healing in the wound fluid and are thought to have a life span of months to years.

— Mast cells: specialized, secretory cells that are important in the inflammatory process.

- At rest contain granules that are a heparin-protein complex that serve as histamine binding sites.
- Contain neutrophil and eosinophil chemotactic factor.
- Release histamine initially after injury to induce temporary mild edema.
- Produces heparin to stimulate migration of endothelial cells.

— Dermal vasculature: two plexuses:

- The upper between papillary and reticular regions which is most of the skin's microcirculation.
- Lower plexus at the reticular dermis and subcutaneous junction.
- Vessels passing vertically between them connect both.
- Dermal lymph vessels drain into larger vessels in the subcutaneous tissue where they acquire valves to ensure one way flow of lymph.
- Thermoregulation

— Behavioral: cold or heat are unpleasant sensations and people will add or delete clothing or seek a change in the environment.

— Physiological: brain centers maintain core body temperature close to 98.6°F.

— Slight elevations in core temperature cause dilation of dermal vessels which causes sweating.

  ▪ Dilation dissipates heat into the environment especially from hands, feet, nose, lips, and ears. The sweating delivers fluid to the skin surface where it evaporates taking off 580 calories per gram.

— Decreases in core body temperature

  ▪ Cause generalized vasoconstriction and blood is shunted away from the skin thereby reducing heat loss.

  ▪ This signals the adrenal glands to increase the metabolic rate of cells and generates heat.

  ▪ The brain centers activate the shivering response that further increases body heat production.

  ▪ Senses

— Dermis contains free and encapsulated nerve endings.

  ▪ Free nerve endings translate sense of heat, cold, pain, and itchiness.

  ▪ Encapsulated nerve endings translate mechanical forces into sense of touch and pressure.

  ▪ Appendages: hair follicles, sweat glands

  ▪ Pilosebaceous apparatus is made up of the hair follicle and sebaceous gland.

  ▪ Hair

  ▪ Hormonal and genetic variations create the individual differences for type, density, rate of growth, color, distribution, pattern, and changes over time.

— Two types of hair:

  ▪ Terminal: scalp hair

  ▪ Vellus: fine, soft hair in "hairless" areas of the body.

■ Melanocytes transfer pigment to growing hair.

■ Hair follicles orient at an angle to the surface of the skin and elevate when the arrector pili muscles contract.

■ Each hair follicle has a sebaceous gland that secretes sebum in response to hormones.

   ○ Sebum is an oily substance that moisturizes the skin and has some immunological properties as well.

— Sweat glands: two types:

  1. Eccrine: tubular structure that secretes water and electrolytes in response to body temperature elevations.

    ○ Each eccrine gland has a duct that opens onto the skin surface.

  2. Apocrine: small in number compared to eccrine glands.

    ○ Limited distribution, larger, deeper in the dermis than eccrine glands.

    ○ Primarily in axillae and anogenital regions.

    ○ Empty into a hair follicle close to skin surface and secretions are mixed with sebum.

• Subcutaneous

• Known as subcutis or hypodermis.

• Thickness varies; dependent on over/under nourishment.

• Contains:

— Loose connective tissue

— Adipose tissue

— Peripheral vascular elements

• Stores about 50% of body's fat: for thermal insulation and a calorie storage depot.

• Principle cells:

— Fibroblasts

— Fat cells

— Macrophages

EFFECTS OF AGING ON SKIN

The skin changes as an individual ages resulting in some changes that create more vulnerability to disease. It is important to recognize and plan care around these changes.

- Dermal-epidermal junction flattens.
- Decreased nutritional flow between layers.
- Reduced resistance to shearing forces that separate the two layers.
- Decrease in skin volume especially in the dermis.
- Decrease in:
  — Connective tissue
  — Vascular elements
  — Sweat glands
  — Sense receptors
  — Cell populations

- Conversion from terminal to vellus hair
  — Generalized graying and loss of hair

- Localized increase in melanin creating age spots to appear although there is a general decrease in number and activity of melanocytes.
- Decreased rate of epidermal turnover
- Decreased rate of wound repair
- Decreased collagen deposition
- Decrease in sweat and sebum production
- Less efficient thermoregulation
- Decreased receptivity of sensory stimuli
- Increased tendency to develop skin growths, benign and malignant
- Collagen and elastin change causing a progressive loss of elastic recovery and decreased extensibility (increases risk of pressure causing skin lesions).

PATIENT HISTORY

Evaluate for specific symptoms of integumentary disease:

- Rash or skin lesion:
  - Onset time: sudden or gradual?
  - Recurrence and location?
  - Initial description of rash or lesion: flat, raised, or blistered?
  - Changes in character over time: new areas involved since it began?
  - Presence of itching, burning, tenderness, pain, numbness, and exudate?
  - Characteristics, bleeding, and color changes?
  - Does sunlight have any effect—aggravate symptoms?
  - Do heat and cold aggravate or improve symptoms?
  - What makes symptoms better or worse?
  - What treatment efforts have been made? When? For how long? Patient response, especially to skin medications?
  - Are cultural healers involved?
  - Any joint pains, fever, fatigue?
  - Has anyone with a similar rash or lesion been in contact or the near patient?
  - Has the patient traveled recently? Where, when, length of stay, exposure to diseases, and any contact with other travelers?
  - History of recent trauma such as falls?
  - Any exposure to a different environment such as the ocean?
  - History of allergy? What are the symptoms?
  - What chronic health problems exist?
- Current medications
  - Aspirin, aspirin-containing medications, over-the-counter medications, and prescriptions?
  - How long has the patient been taking the medication?
  - Describe recent changes in medications or any recent injections received.

— Any recreational or illicit drug use? What drugs? How long using these drugs? Route of administration?

  ■ A sudden reaction to medications used for years is not uncommon.

— Describe use of soaps, deodorants, cosmetics, colognes, household products, latex, and sunscreens. Any changes in use of these in last few weeks or months?

  ■ Manufacturers may change formulas at any time without notifying the consumer.

• Contributing factors
  — Patient's occupation or avocation
  — Recreational activities
  — Alcohol use
  — Menses history
  — Gardening, household repairs, or contact with animals
    ■ May reveal exposure to chemicals or similar agents
  — Specific food allergies or changes
  — Recent visitors such as young children?
  — Recent physiologic stress?
  — Family history of similar skin disorders, infestations, asthma, or hay fever?
  — Psychogenic factors that may contribute to skin condition?
  — Nutritional habits?
  — Patient and caregiver's perception of cause and treatment?
  — How are patient and caregiver adjusting to skin condition?
  — History of skin self-exam?

• Changes in skin color, texture, turgor, and temperature
  — Onset time: sudden or gradual?
  — Recurrence and location?
  — Initial description, changes over time, localized or generalized?
  — Normal skin color is ebony to porcelain and every shade in between

— Often darker in intertriginous areas, male genitalia, peri-anal skin, areolae, and following sun exposure.

— Dark skinned persons may have a bluish tinge to the nailbeds and lips.

— Heat, excitement, or embarrassment may cause a dull to bright red flush in the skin of the face and upper torso.

— This may also be induced by hormonally controlled vascular instability of perimenopausal "hotflashes."

• Current medications

— Aspirin, aspirin-containing medications, over-the-counter medications, and prescriptions?

— How long has the patient been taking the medication?

— Describe recent changes in medications or any recent injections received.

— Any recreational or illicit drug use? What drugs? How long using these drugs? Route of administration?

  ▪ A sudden reaction to medications used for years is not uncommon.

• Texture

— Assessment questions as above.

— Variable in normal persons.

— Sun-exposed areas are drier and coarser than protected areas unless moisturized at least daily.

— Aging skin is often thinner and more transparent than younger skin.

• Characteristics of melanoma

— Asymmetry: borders that are irregular rather than smooth with scalloped edges, notches, pseudopods, or satellite foci of pigment discontinuous with a specific lesion.

— Color: very deeply pigmented or highly variable pigmentation; deep brown, black, highly variegated, red-white-and-blue, or areas of depigmentation.

— Diameter: over 6 mm in greatest dimension.

- Cancer risk factors
  — Age older than 50 years
  — Male
  — Fair, freckled, or ruddy complexion
  — Light-colored hair or eyes
  — Tendency to burn easily
  — Overexposure to frost, wind, or ultraviolet B radiation from the sun
  — Geographic location near the equator or high altitudes
  — Exposure to arsenic, creosote, coal tar, or petroleum products
  — Family history of cancer
  — Overexposure to radium, radioisotopes, x-rays, repeated trauma, or irritation to skin
  — History of precancerous dermatoses
- Turgor
  — Assessment questions as above
  — Varies due to hydration and age
  — Age causes alteration in elastin in dermis which may create tenting.
- Temperature
  — Assessment questions as above
  — Related to ambient room temperature, core body temperature, and autonomic (emotional) responses to the environment.
  — Not necessarily abnormal to have cool hands or feet.
  — Consider the entire clinical picture when assessing temperature.
- Pruritus
  — Onset time: sudden or gradual?
  — Recurrence and location?
  — Initial description, changes over time, localized or generalized?

— Any changes in sweating or dryness of body?

— Does sunlight have any effect—aggravate symptoms?

— Do heat and cold aggravate or improve symptoms?

— What makes symptoms better or worse?

— What treatment efforts have been made? When? For how long? Patient response, especially to skin medications?

— Are cultural healers involved?

• Current medications

— Aspirin, aspirin-containing medications, over-the-counter medications, and prescriptions?

— How long has the patient been taking the medication?

— Describe recent changes in medications or any recent injections received.

— Any recreational or illicit drug use? What drugs? How long using these drugs? Route of administration?

  ▪ A sudden reaction to medications used for years is not uncommon

— Describe use of soaps, deodorants, cosmetics, colognes, household products, latex, and sunscreens. Any changes in use of these in last few weeks or months?

  ▪ Manufacturers may change formulas at any time without notifying the consumer.

• Contributing factors

— Patient's occupation or avocation

— Recreational activities

— Alcohol use

— Menses history

— Gardening, household repairs, or contact with animals

  ▪ May reveal exposure to chemicals or similar agents

— Specific food allergies or changes

— Recent visitors such as young children?

— Recent physiologic stress?

— Family history of similar skin disorders, infestations, asthma, or hay fever?

— Psychogenic factors that may contribute to skin condition?

— Nutritional habits?

— Has the patient traveled recently? Where, when, length of stay, exposure to diseases, and any contact with other travelers?

— History of allergy? What are the symptoms?

— What chronic health problems exist?

   ▪ Diffuse prorates are often observed in biliary cirrhosis, dermatitis herpetiformis, and cancer, especially lymphoma. This may also be a symptom of aging, which can be dealt with by daily moisturization. Or, it may be one of the first signs of medication allergy.

- Changes in hair

— Onset time: sudden or gradual?

— Recurrence and location?

— Initial description, changes over time, localized or generalized?

— Unusual growth or distribution?

— Brittleness or breakage?

— Associated with any rash, lesion, itching, fever, or recent stress?

— Any exposure to toxins or commercial hair preparations?

— Changes in care of hair?

— Changes in diet?

— What makes symptoms better or worse?

— What efforts are being taken to treat the hair? When? For how long? Response to medications, especially hair loss medications?

— Cultural healers consulted?

— Ask the same questions about medications as in the sections above.

— Any thyroid or liver disorders?

— Severe illness or malnutrition?

— Frequent causes of hair loss are aging and loss of hormones and changes in diet, medications, and hair care products.

— Hypothyroidism causes loss of the lateral third of eyebrows.

— Vascular (arterial) disease causes hair loss on legs.

— Hair loss also occurs in heavy metal poisoning, hypopituitarism, or nutritional states such as pellagra.

— Ovarian and adrenal tumors may cause an increase in body hair.

— In aging, hair texture becomes finer and axillary and pubic hair may be thin or lost.

• Changes in nails

— Onset time: sudden or gradual?

— Recurrence and location?

— Initial description, changes over time, localized or generalized?

— Unusual growth or distribution?

— Brittleness or breakage?

— Associated with any rash, lesion, or other skin condition?

— History of congenital anomalies or respiratory, cardiac, endocrine, hematologic, or other systemic disease?

— Nail color varies with general skin pigmentation.

— Dark-skinned individuals may have visible darkly pigmented bands in the nails.

— Longitudinal ridging and shallow pits are normal variants.

— Tobacco smokers may have yellow-brown staining from nicotine in the fingers that hold the tobacco product.

— Subungual hematomas are often secondary to hemorrhage beneath the nail caused by trauma.

— Ingrown nails, especially of the toes, present as swollen, inflamed paronchia at the distal corners.

- General assessment questions
  - Always ask about changes in moles, birthmarks, or other body spots.
  - Assess for color changes, irregular growth, pain, scaling, or bleeding.
  - Are there any red, scaly, or crusted areas of the skin that do not heal?
  - Ask if the patient has ever had skin cancer?
  - Ask about the location of the cancer and treatment?
  - Any recent growth of a flat, pigmented lesion is relevant information.

PHYSICAL EXAMINATION

When arranging the visit by telephone, request that the patient wear loose clothing that is easy to remove. For the examination have the patient seated in a comfortable position and wearing loose clothing. Be certain there is a good light source. This may be the closest window during daylight hours with window treatments open. Tangential lighting will assist with assessing contour (e.g., from a flashlight). Generally, the skin is inspected during the assessment of other body systems; however, be certain that the skin assessment and evaluation are thorough.

- Inspect
  - All areas not usually exposed such as axillae, buttocks, perineum, backs of thighs, inner upper thighs, feet, and intertriginous surfaces.
  - In the individual with a darker complexion the best areas to determine actual color are sclera, conjunctiva, buccal mucosa, tongue, lips, nail beds, and palms.
  - Normal variation may include opaque yellow color in heavily calloused palms or soles, lighter palms and soles, hyperpigmented macules on soles, and freckling in the buccal cavity, gums, and tongue.

— The sclera may have a "muddy" appearance or brownish pigment that looks like petechiae.

— A bluish hue to the lips and gums may also be a normal finding.

— Remember that systemic disorders may cause generalized or localized color changes.

— Localized redness may be due to an inflammatory process.

— Pale, shiny skin on the lower extremities may be due to peripheral changes from diabetes mellitus or cardiovascular disease.

— Localized hemorrhages into cutaneous tissues may be from injury, steroids, vasculitis, or systemic disorders.

— If a red-purple discoloration is caused by injury it is called ecchymoses; if caused by other factors and less than 0.5 cm it is called petechiae; if larger than 0.5 cm in diameter it is called purpura.

Hair

• Distribution and texture: commonly present on scalp, lower face, neck, nares, ears, chest, axillae, back, shoulders, arms, legs, toes, pubic area, and around nipples.

• Quantity and color

• Dryness or brittleness

• Lesions or crusts

• Hair loss general or localized

— Loss on feet and/or toes may indicate poor circulation or nutritional deficit.

• Inflammation or scarring with hair loss

• Hair shafts broken off or completely absent

• Alopecia or hirsutism

• Cleanliness and general scalp and hair condition including patient self-care ability.

Nails

- Shape
- Cleanliness including patient self-care ability
- Symmetry
- General configuration
- Color; thickness; shape; peeling
- Brittleness
- Smooth, rounded nail edges
- Hemorrhages under the nail
- Transverse lines or grooves in nail or nail bed: can indicate repeated nail injury or chronic manipulation
- Spoon nails: koilonchia indicates iron deficiency anemia
- Beau lines: transverse grooves parallel to the lunula associated with significant infections and renal or hepatic diseases
- Clubbing: the base angle should measure 160° with a firm nail bed; can indicate cardiac, pulmonary, or cystic fibrosis causes
- Pitting can indicate psoriasis
- Hyperkeratosis can be caused by fungus, bacteria, or aging
- Proximal and lateral nail folds should be inspected for redness, swelling, pus, warts, cysts, or tumors.
- Lindsay nails: proximal nail bed with white, red, or pink can indicate chronic renal disease or hypoalbuminemia
- Terry nails: white nail beds with 1 mm to 2 mm distal nail border can indicate cirrhosis or hypoalbuminemia

Face and Neck

- Solar elastosis: deep furrows in neck and face skin; assess for more threatening sun damage
- Skin tags, soft polyps, or normal looking and feeling skin

Breasts, axillae, and chest

- Inframammary dermatitis: superficial mycosis in intertriginous breast or axillary folds; chronicity can produce pustules and hyperpigmentation

- Symmetry, ulcerations, orange peel texture, pulling or pitting of breast tissue
- Hidradenitis suppurativa: recurrent infection of sweat glands with significant erythema; chronicity leads to scarring
- Skin tags
- Herpes zoster: distribution along spinal or cranial nerves; vesicular eruptions and bullae on erythematous bases with pain

Abdomen

- Intertriginous folds condition
- Grey Turner sign: flank discoloration
- Cullen sign: periumbilical blueness seen with pancreatitis, peritoneal dialysis causing peritonitis, and splenic rupture from infectious mononucleosis
- Condition of scars: often abnormal in patients with defective healing such as diabetics; hyperpigmentation; keloid

Back

- Pressure areas
- Fluid collection areas
- Pilonidal cyst
- Moles
- Growths

Perianal Area

- External hemorrhoids: gray-blue to flesh-colored masses near the anal verge; can be thrombotic and painful
- Fissures-in-ano: tender, linear breaks in perianal skin painful with defecation or manipulation; larger, ragged, inflamed defects are often indicative of Crohn disease

Genitalia

- Genital herpes simplex: tiny vesicles with erythematous bases and severe pain often preceding the physical sign
- Genital warts

- Condylomata acuminata: from infection with human papilloma virus (HPV); usually small, white-pink, and often clustered on penis, vulva, perineum, scrotum, or anal region. May also be systemic and some strains cause cancer of vulva, penis, and uterine cervix
- Vulvar dystrophy: discoloration often macular or patch-like, overt skin atrophy or fine wrinkling. Common in postreproductive ages some are associated with increased cancer risk.

Lower Extremities

- Epithelial defects
- Medial malleolus: venous ulcer
- Hemosiderin deposits: venous insufficiency
- Diabetic shin spots: sunken brownish spots over anterior skins

Feet

- General condition: dry, flaking, fissured, calloused, or ulcerated
- Assess the skin between the toes
- Tinea pedis (athlete's foot): pruritus, tenderness, and desquamation of white epithelium with scant exudate. May be a precursor or cause of cellulitis as a result of streptococci.
- Gangrene: dry or wet

Expected Skin Findings in Older Adults

- Cherry angiomas: tiny ruby red, round papules that become brown over time; occur at age 30 and increase in numbers with age
- Seborrheic keratoses: pigmented, wart-like, raised lesions usually on face or trunk
- Sebaceous hyperplasia: yellow, flat papules with central depressions
- Cutaneous tags: small, soft, usually on neck and upper chest; may be pedunculated (attached to body by a narrow stalk); may or may not be pigmented
- Cutaneous horns: small, hard projections of epidermis most often on the forehead or face

- Senile lentigines: irregular, round, gray-brown lesions with rough surface; most common in sun-exposed areas "age or liver spots"

Palpation

- Skin surfaces
  — Moisture
  — Temperature
  — Texture
  — Turgor
  — Mobility
- Nail plates
  — Normal is hard, smooth, firm with uniform thickness and adherence to nail bed; thickening may result from tight-fitting shoes, chronic trauma, or fungal infections
  — Pain in nail groove may be secondary to ischemia
  — Separation of nail plate from bed: psoriasis, *Candida*, *Pseudomonas* infection, some medications, or trauma
- Periwound area
  — Induration
  — Pain
  — Temperature
  — Increased exudate
- Hair
  — Texture

APPLICATION AND REMOVAL OF ADHESIVES TO SKIN

Application:

- Assess for latex or other adhesive allergies before application.
- Most adhesives require skin to be thoroughly cleansed and dried before application or the skin tac will not adhere.

- Use a picture frame adhesive technique when the intent is to create as complete a barrier to outside forces as possible (or a dressing that is occlusive such as Tegaderm or Tegasorb).

- An "H"— three, or more stripe pattern of adhesive may be used to secure dressings if such a barrier is not necessary.

- When applying adhesive to any usually moist surface such as the perianal area it is most effective to prepare the area with a skin barrier wipe (such as 3M No Sting) first; allow this to dry thoroughly before adhesive application.

Removal:

- Thorough assessment of the dressing and appliance before removal is part of professional evaluation.

- Use a "push the skin gently away from the adhesive" while "pulling the adhesive away from the skin" technique with all adhesives.

  — This technique creates the least amount of skin damage.

  — Whenever it is appropriate for the patient to shower immediately before the adhesive removal, have him or her do so. This will moisten the adhesive and therefore adhere less aggressively at the time of removal.

  — If using adhesive removal products it is important to gently, thoroughly cleanse all adhesive remover from the skin. Most of these products leave some residue on the skin that may cause a chemical reaction or create a nonadherent surface.

General Guidelines for Adhesive Use:

- Use the least amount of adhesive necessary to keep the dressing or appliance in place for the most therapeutic time.

- Use nonadhesive products to secure the dressings whenever possible such as Montgomery straps and stretch bandages.

- Use barrier wipes under the adhesives whenever the patient has fragile skin or the dressing or appliance requires changing more than once or twice every 5 to 7 days and as clinically necessary.

- Document the clinical rationale for the use of supplemental products with adhesives such as barrier wipes and stretch bandages.

DOCUMENTATION

- The complete assessment and evaluation should be documented.
- Each wound should be defined by type of wound (trauma, pressure ulcer, venous ulcer, arterial ulcer, or surgical wound) for reimbursement purposes and stage if a pressure ulcer. It cannot be categorized as both a pressure ulcer and a diabetic ulcer although the presence of diabetes may impact the healing rate of the pressure ulcer.
- The wound requires a diagnosis from a provider whose level of practice indicates their ability with diagnosing.
- Each wound should be coded according to wound type and procedure that is performed. For example, pressure ulcer stage III with surgical debridement. Codes may be found in the ICDM for diagnoses and in the CPT coding for procedures. Additional information may be obtained from the American Health Information Management Association (AHIMA) (http://www.ahima.org/).

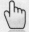 **Nursing Note**
- *If the wound is of a surgical nature the date of the surgery must be indicated in the initial evaluation of the patient.*
- *If the wound is of a traumatic nature the date of the initial trauma and the type of trauma must be indicated in the initial evaluation of the patient.*
- *In a surgical or trauma wound, it is helpful to also document the type of treatment the patient has received since the beginning of treatment and whether this has created healing in the wound.*

- Each wound should be classified according to the depth of tissue involved from the epidermis downward.
  — Intact skin
  — Superficial
  — Partial thickness
  — Full thickness
- Surgical wounds: an acute surgical wound is generally categorized as healing according to the preoperative expectations of healing time, and chronic surgical wounds are all those which do not.
  — Acute
  — Chronic
- Nonsurgical wounds: an acute nonsurgical wound is generally categorized as healing according to the expectations of usual healing time for the particular wound type, and chronic nonsurgical wounds are all those which do not.
  — Acute
  — Chronic
- Document the cause of the wound whenever it is known. For example, patient states, "I bumped it into the trash can lid about 2 weeks ago and this wound has been getting bigger ever since."

 Nursing Alert
All documentation should be consistent with the treatment plan and the expected outcome.

- All encounters with the patient should be documented even if they are telephone or electronic messaging in nature.
- Wound shape and size
  — Wound size: measure wounds as if they were on the face of a clock with the head of patient at 12:00; the feet of the patient at 6:00; the right arm at 9:00; and the left arm at 3:00 (Figure 10–1).

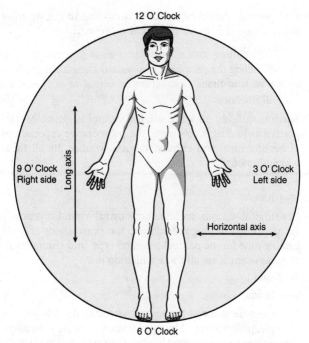

Figure 10–1 Wound Size. (Adapted with permission from Baranoski S, Ayello E. *Wound Care Essentials Practice Principles.* Philadelphia, PA: Lippincott Williams & Wilkins; 2004.)

— Describe the overall wound shape: oval, elliptical, or irregular
— Wound length in centimeters with length according to patient head to foot location
— Wound width in centimeters with width according to patient arm to arm location
— Wound depth (may vary throughout the wound) in centimeters

— Wound edges or margins: rolled, punched out, irregular, or macerated

— Undermining: tissue destruction extending under intact skin along the periphery of a wound or tunneling; course or path of tissue destruction occurring in any direction from the surface or edge of the wound; results in dead space with potential for abscess formation; may have both at the same time.

- Tissue type and amount
  — The amount should indicate the percent of the wound bed and edges that are of a specific tissue type. For example: 50% granulation tissue and 50% thin, yellow, fibrous slough.
  — Granulation
  — Slough
  — Eschar
- Exudate
  — Amount on the dressing within 24 hours or since the last dressing change; indicate when the last dressing change occurred.
  — Color: serous, sero-sanguinous, or purulent
  — Odor: none, mild, or foul
  — Consistency: thin or thick
- Surrounding or periwound skin
  — Intact
  — Macerated
  — Erythematous
- Stage of pressure ulcers
  — Stage I
  — Stage II
  — Stage III
  — Stage IV
  — Unstageable

> **Nursing Alert**
> *All wounds other than neuropathic or diabetic are documented as partial or full thickness.*
> *Remember that pressure ulcers may heal but are always documented by the deepest amount of tissue involved. Therefore, a stage III pressure ulcer is always a stage III pressure ulcer and is documented as a healing stage III unless the wound worsens to a stage IV. There is currently no back or down-staging of pressure ulcers during healing.*

- Document the current treatment, the patient's ability to adhere to the treatment plan, and any changes in the treatment plan with rationale for these changes.
- Document patient and caregiver education provided including their ability to state the education in their own words and their intention of doing as the education suggests. For example: elevate your left leg above heart level every 2 hours throughout the day for at least 15 minutes each time. Patient states, "I will elevate my leg on a pillow every 2 hours for 15 minutes during the day at work."
- Document the patient's pain level at dressing change or treatment and during the time between dressing changes or treatments. It is recommended to use a scale that begins with no or zero pain and goes up in increments to the worst pain ever experienced. There are a variety of pain scales that have been validated with differing patient populations.
  - Documentation must include what the health-care provider has done about the patient's pain. This must include whether the action has produced the desired effect or not.
  - Document what actions the patient has taken to alleviate the pain and whether these have achieved any difference in pain level. For example: "I lowered my leg over the bed and after about 15 minutes it was tolerable."
- When removing the dressing, note the condition of the dressing and document this in the medical record. For example:

primary dressing 50% saturated in 24 hours with serous exudates without odor.

- At each patient encounter provide the patient with 'homework'—something to do before the next encounter. For example: patient will note the number of times he performs ankle pump exercises and will discuss success with these at next encounter.
- Documentation of durable medical equipment (DME)
  — Type of equipment ordered and rationale. For example: non-powered mattress to redistribute pressure on trunk and buttocks at site of pressure ulcer
  — Education of patient and caregiver received regarding:
    - Name and rationale for device
    - Who to call if the device fails or requires maintenance
    - What to do with device if patient encounters an emergency such as a natural disaster
    - Actions to take if patient no longer requires the device for treatment. This may be if the patient is hospitalized or if the wound is healed.
    - Party responsible for the maintenance of the device
    - Party responsible for keeping the device clean
- Documentation regarding medical supplies such as dressings
  — Education of patient and caregiver regarding:
    - Party responsible for ordering appropriate amounts of medical supplies
    - How and when to order medical supplies
    - How to properly store medical supplies in locations other than a hospital or clinic
    - When to refer to other providers and what to document

REFERRAL TO SPECIALTY NURSES, PHYSICIANS, AND OTHER DISCIPLINES

Purpose:

- Provide the level of care necessitated by the patient's clinical needs.

- Provide support and expertise to the clinician or provider.
- Ensure that each patient receives appropriate levels and types of wound care and other health-care services through provider utilization.
- Serve as evidence of individualization of care.

Timing (when to refer to whom):

- The wound has not progressed in a specific period of time or as expected, usually 10 to 14 days of treatment.
  — Physician when orders are required or a consult or visit is needed
  — Certified Wound Ostomy Continence Nurse/Enterostomal Therapy Nurse (CWOCN/ET nurse)

  OR
  — Clinical Nurse Specialist (CNS) if available

  OR
  — Nursing supervisor
  — Registered Dietitian (RD) if full thickness or prealbumin or serum albumin are below normal levels
- The wound is not responding to appropriate treatment in a specific period of time or as expected.
  — Physician when orders are required or a consult/visit is needed
  — CWOCN/ET nurse

  OR
  — CNS (if available)

  OR
  — Nursing supervisor
  — RD if full thickness or prealbumin or serum albumin are below normal levels
  — The clinical provider has questions concerning the treatment, the expected wound healing process, or expected outcomes.
    ▪ Individual who wrote or requested the orders for wound care or the plan of care (POC).

- The clinical provider requires assistance in managing a particularly challenging wound, patient, caregiver, and situation.
  — CWOCN/ET/CNS
    - Wound care is not effective in expected time period.
    - Products are not efficacious, too difficult for patient or caregiver to manage, too expensive, or not available.
    - Required wound care can only be provided by CWOCN as in the case of conservative or sharp debridement.
    - Questions concerning type and amount of pressure reduction devices.
  — MSW: to evaluate the patient or caregiver who is unwilling or unable to participate in the wound care as developed in the POC.
    - Request the MSW to determine if there are any psychological or sociological reasons for this inability or unwillingness.
    - Request the MSW to assist in developing a POC for all other providers to reach the expected and planned for outcomes. This includes a plan to manage health and other patient/caregiver behaviors.
    - Request MSW to assist when there are financial concerns of the patient or caregiver relative to the POC such as the ability to pay copayments.
  — Occupational Therapist (OT)
    - Whenever there is a question about the patient or caregiver's potential for self-care of the wound or independence in other activities of daily living (ADLs).
    - When there are questions concerning the amount of energy conservation needed in a specific situation.
    - When there are questions concerning adaptive equipment to further the patient's independence.
  — Physical Therapy (PT)
    - Whenever there are questions concerning the patient's mobility and independent function relative to mobility.

- ▪ Whenever the patient or caregiver requires education regarding independence with mobility devices such as transfer boards.
— Registered Dietitian (RD)
  - ▪ When the prealbumin or serum albumin are below normal.
  - ▪ The patient is receiving enteral or parenteral nutrition.
  - ▪ The patient is on a "special" diet such as a renal or vegan diet.
  - ▪ The wound is full thickness or there are multiple wounds.

SUGGESTED READING

Diegelmann R, Parks W, Harding K. Research: Pathophysiology of Wound Epithelization. Paper presented at 2003 Symposium on Advanced Wound Care, April 28, 2003, Las Vegas, NV.

Langemo DK, et al. The lived experiences of having a pressure ulcer: a qualitative analysis. *Advances in Skin and Wound Care.* Sept–Oct. 2000;13(5):225–235.

Petro J. Ethical and psychosocial considerations of wound management. *Decubitus.* January 1992;5(1):22–25.

Price P. Defining and measuring quality of life. *Journal of Wound Care.* March 1996;5(3):139–140.

Renberger K. Can't we just agree: exploring the ethics of identifying goals of care or cure. Paper presented at 2003 Wound, Ostomy, and Continence Nurses Society 35th Annual Conference, June 16, 2003, Cincinnati, OH.

Schipper H, et al. Quality of life studies: definitions and conceptual issues. In: *Quality of life and Pharmacoeconomics in Clinical Trials.* 2nd ed. Ed, Spilker B., Philadelphia, PA: Lippincott-Raven; 1996.

Seidel H, Ball J, Dains J, Benedict GW. *Mosby's Guide to Physical Examination.* 4th ed. St Louis, MO: Mosby Inc; 1999.

Sussman C, Bates-Jensen B. *Wound Care A Collaborative Practice Manual for Physical Therapists and Nurses.* Gaithersburg, MD: Aspen Publications; 1998.

Support Systems International, Inc. *The Skin, Module 1*. Charleston, SC: Hillenbrand; 1993.

Swartz M. *Textbook of Physical Diagnosis History and Examination*. 3rd ed. Philadelphia, PA: WB Saunders; 1998.

Tierney L, McPhee S, Papadakis M. *Current Medical Diagnosis and Treatment*. 37th ed. Stamford, CT: Appleton & Lange;1998.

Index

Page numbers followed by *f* or *t* indicate figures or tables, respectively.